How to Master the USMLE Step 1:
Askdoc's Method of USMLE Prep

First Edition

MIKE NICOL UY, M.D.

DEDICATION

This book is dedicated to my parents, Richard and Soledad, without whom I would not be here.

Table of Contents

ACKNOWLEDGMENTS

I would like to acknowledge my assistant Meliza Tadena for the invaluable help she gave to make this book a reality.

unit 1

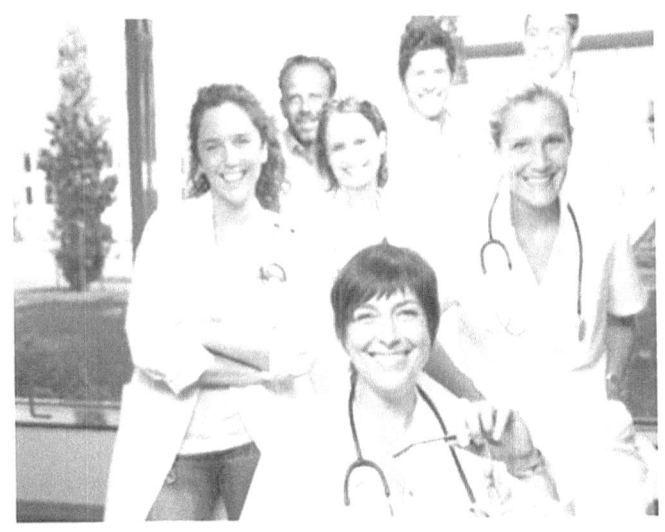

Master the USMLE Step 1

CHAPTER 1
WHY YOU NEED TO MASTER THE USMLE STEP 1?

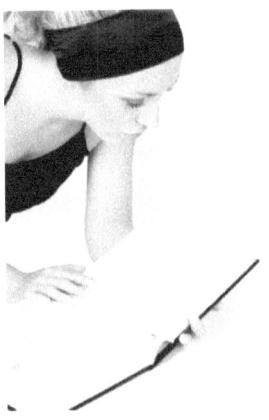

Factors to Consider

Taking the USMLE is different from any exam you have ever taken before. If you are an IMG, chances are it is different from the board exam you took in your home country. Therefore, you need to take into account those features that can affect your performance in the USMLE and adjust for them during your prep. For an AMG, the length of the exam, the sheer amount of details you need to read and memorize and the emphasis on analysis and understanding mechanisms rather than just memorizing facts can be quite daunting. Therefore it makes sense that you would take more time and effort to prepare for the USMLE than for other exams.

Everyone has a Limited Memory Capacity

Unless you have photographic memory, you can't remember everything. Everyone has a limited memory capacity. That is true for you, for me, for those who have failed the exams and for those who aced it. Different people have different memory capacities. Some may be larger, others smaller, but in the end, our memory capacities are limited. This is probably the single biggest reason why we need to prep properly in the first place. If we have unlimited memory, we can just open a book and start reading. By the time you finish the nth book, you know and can remember everything you need to ace the exam. But because of this limitation, it's not possible to do it that way and you need to take that into consideration in your prep. Later, we will discuss ways to increase the amount of information we can store in our limited memories. It requires some work and you will need to study a certain way in order to take advantage of it. But, it is doable.

USMLE Coverage is just too broad

The USMLE website has a list of all the topics that may come out in the exam. If you actually studied everything listed there, you will realize that you need to study all the major textbooks of each of the subjects covered and journals published in the past 5 years. It is impossible to study everything. Therefore, deciding what you are going to study and how detailed you are going to study them is a very important step in your preparation.

There are two things we need to understand though. First, with just over 300 questions in Step 1, the USMLE cannot cover everything. Therefore, you know you do not need to study everything. Second, the USMLE has a mandate, and that is to ensure that medical students have the necessary basic and clinical science knowledge in medicine to practice safely and effectively. Knowing this, we have an idea of what medical topics have the best chance of coming out in the exam. We need to focus on them and make sure we cover them thoroughly.

You start forgetting almost immediately after you start reading

The minute you finished reading the first chapter of Pathology, you start forgetting almost immediately what you have read. That is true for you, for me, for people who failed, who passed and who got a 99. Worse if you studied anything in between, you forget even more since the new information will tend to crowd out the old one.

For example, two weeks after reading chapter 1 of pathology, you would have forgotten some of what you have studied. But if you read chapter 2 of pathology in the interim, you would have forgotten even more of chapter 1 than if you have not read anything in between.

Therefore, you can understand how big a problem this can be in the USMLE. The amount of materials you need to study and the length of time needed to cover those materials can make it very difficult to retain and recall the information you have studied. Although we can't entirely stop the forgetting process, there are specific study methods that can help in minimizing this forgetting process. We will discuss them in detail in a while.

You have a limited time to study

You can't study forever. For medical students, they may need to take the examination by a certain date as part of the requirement of their medical school. Even for IMG's who can actually take the examination anytime they want, they can't study too long or risk burning out. Therefore, there is a need to plan out your prep so you can finish studying all you have to cover on time and do well in the examination.

Whereas some people approach the USMLE as if they have all the time in the world to prepare for it, there are some of those on the other hand, that give themselves too little time to cover all they need to do properly. Remember you don't just need to read about these topics. You need to read, understand, correlate, integrate, memorize and recall all these topics. And you need to be able to recall them fast at the right level of detail to be able to answer the questions properly. This requires more preparation than what you need for a short quiz or even for a shelf exam.

The USMLE is a time-limited exam

A big reason why the USMLE is so tough is because your time to answer the questions is so limited. Given enough time, most people can score rather high in the examination. Therefore, you need to be able to read fast, recall fast and analyze even faster to do well in this exam. You need to take that into account in your prep. There are study methods that will help you with this and we will discuss them in more detail later.

The USMLE is a very long exam

The USMLE Step 1 is an 8 hour exam composed of 7 blocks of 46 questions each. You have 1 hour to accomplish each block for a total of 7 hours plus 1 hour of total breaks for the day. This requires a level of stamina that most people tend to underestimate. When you are hitting the 5th or 6th block, your brain is tired. You need to read questions twice to understand them. It takes longer for you to recall information. It takes even longer to find the answer. Some questions you could have easily answered if only you encountered it in your first block, you find you are unable to answer because it's in the 5th block. In short your brain has turned to mush and that's part of what makes USMLE tough.

Therefore there is a need to account for this in the exam. When you do your online q banks or your NBME, you are doing it in the relative comfort of the library or your house, doing at most 4 blocks straight. Therefore, expecting the same level of performance on all 7 blocks in the actual exam is a bit naive. If you are just barely passing when you are fresh, imagine what is happening on the 6th and 7th blocks when your brain is tired and refusing to work. That is why it is imperative that you over study and score higher in the q banks and NBME than the minimum needed to pass. This will give you the buffer you need to insure that you will get the score you want on the day of the exam. Training to increase your stamina will also help.

You need to be able to recall what you have studied

For the purpose of the USMLE, what you cannot recall, you do not know. This is where a lot of people make their mistake when studying for the USMLE. They think all they need to do is study and memorize the medical concepts and that is enough. Worse, some people even think that all they need is to understand the concepts and they are all good.

A lot of times during the examination, I can't recall a specific topic, but immediately after finishing the block, everything comes flashing back in my head. I had studied and memorize the information but I have a hard time recalling the information. Therefore, it is important that as part of your prep, you not only study and memorize but practice recalling the information very fast. Again there are various study methods to improve recall and they are not the same as those that help you memorize and retain information. We'll discuss them in more detail in the section on How to Study. ■

CHAPTER 2

WHAT YOU NEED TO KNOW IN ORDER TO DO WELL IN THE USMLE STEP 1?

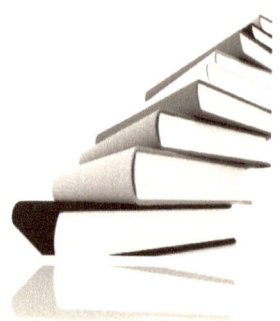

First, you need to know what to study. Second, you need to know how much to study and lastly, you need to know how to study.

What to Study?

You need to study the right things. You need to know what to study and what not to study. Studying the wrong things wastes not only your limited time but your limited memory capacity. It can also cause you to fail the exam.

Examples of studying the wrong things, include

- *Studying things that will not come out in the examination.* Don't waste your limited time and memory space studying concepts that will not come out in the exam, spend it instead on studying and remembering concepts that will be tested in the exam. You would be surprised at how many people make this error in their prep. It is possible that you may need to study some things that will not come out in the exam in order to understand things that will come out. But these are exceptions, and you don't need to memorize them in detail, just understand them.

- *Failing to study things that will definitely come out in the exam.* High yield topics are topics that have a very high chance of coming out in the exam. Therefore it is important to make sure you cover all the high yield stuff in your review. A lot of lower yield topics will also come out in the exam, therefore ignoring them completely is not exactly a good idea.

- *Studying at a wrong level of detail for the exam.* The USMLE expects you to know some topics in more detail than others. You need to make sure you study the topics at the level of detail that the USMLE expects or you won't be able to answer the questions. We will discuss this in more detail under Mastery, Know and Familiar.

Most people depend on reviewers to tell them what they need to study. However, reviewers rarely agree with each other what will come out in the examination. If you look at First Aid, Kaplan Notes and BRS, you will note that there is a lot of difference in terms of topic covered. So which of them is right, you may ask --actually all of them. Part of the reason there is a difference in coverage has to do with the original intent of the author. For example, First Aid was primarily written as a high yield review for third year medical students aiming to pass the USMLE and have undergone some form of prep by their medical school. Usually, the knowledge is still fresh in their head and a short high yield review is all they need to pass this exam. On the other hand, Kaplan notes try to cover more details that will help IMGs who are mostly older graduates. Even for a new grad, basic science is more than two years past and a lot of information is no longer fresh. It also contains enough material to score high in the exam but not ace it. Meanwhile BRS is somewhere between the two extremes.

Therefore, you need to be aware of your current situation and your goals and whether the review material you are using applies to you or help you achieve the goal you are aiming for. Using First Aid when you want a high score can prove fatal to your plans.

How Much to Study?

It is not enough to study the right things; you need to study them in the right level of detail expected in the USMLE. One of the most common question asked by my students is 'Should I memorize the classification of viruses? Should I know whether they are linear, circular or icosahedral, naked or enveloped? Or I know we need to study genetic testing, but do we really need to study how it's done step by step?' The right answer of course depends on the topic. Some topics you need to study in detail, others you don't. We'll discuss this in more detail on the section on Mastery, Know and Familiar.

If you read the forums, you will notice that most people study the same materials and yet the results range from high 99's to failure. One of the main reasons is failing to study in the right amount of detail. You need to know how detailed you need to study in order to achieve a certain score. Not studying enough details can lead to low scores or worse failing even if you are studying the right materials. On the other hand going into too much detail requires time and memory capacity which may be quite limited.

It's not enough to study the right amount of details but to make sure you memorized, retained and be able to recall the right level of detail as well. You may have read and studied the topic at the right level of detail, but if you can recall only half of that detail during the exam, it will not help.

For example, in my prep course, we make it a point to indicate how detailed you need to study to achieve a certain score. If you meet the minimum requirements of the course, on average you will score between 85 to 95. If you put in less than the minimum effort, you will score lower. If you want to get a higher score, you need to supplement your study and will be told by how much. Of course it goes without saying that you have to be able to retain and recall the information at the level of detail presented in the course. You need to know how to study properly in order to insure you are able to do that.

How to Study?

If you go to the forums, you will see that everyone is studying practically the same things. First Aid, Kaplan Notes, BRS, USMLE World Q bank. And yet the results vary from failing to high 99's. One of the main reasons is that people have varying study skills and most people just do not know how to study. If you join most prep courses or buy reviewers to study, they tell you that you need to study, understand, memorize and be able to recall these topics for the exam. It is presumed you know how to do that. But on most cases people don't have enough study skills to do this effectively and efficiently for an exam like the USMLE.

So why do we need to know how to study? Most people are able to survive medical school without knowing how to study. Some people have passable study skills and that is all that is needed to pass medical school. But the USMLE is different from all other exams we have taken in medical school. Most exams we have taken in medical school are short, even the shelf exams for each subject. Anatomy for example. After studying and sitting for your Anatomy Shelf exam, you can start forgetting it when you start studying for the Physiology shelf exam. When it comes to the USMLE, you are expected to remember all 7 subjects which you took 2 years to study in the first place. And you are not allowed to forget anything until that one day you when for 8 long hours you sit for the exam.

Another thing is that for the purpose of the USMLE, what you cannot recall during the exam, you do not know. In fact, what you cannot recall in about a minute or less, you do not know. The USMLE does not care how much you have studied. It does not care how many sleepless nights you have gone through. It does not care how hard you have studied or what books you have read. How many thousands of questions you have answered or how many qbanks you have finished. Nor what sacrifices you have gone through and what emotional turmoil you have undergone. If you cannot answer the question, you do not know it. You don't even get partial points. Unlike in medical school where other factors such as attendance, performance in group reports, etc. counts toward your final score, in the USMLE, the only thing that counts is what happens during the day of the examination. Therefore, all your preparation must make sure that you are at your best on that day.

Lastly, everyone has weak points. Whether it is poor memory, slow reading speed, difficulty with clinical vignettes or difficulty with two to three step thinking questions, everyone has their own weak points. There are specific study methodologies that can address each and every one of these weak points. We may not be able to completely eliminate those weak points, but we can mitigate them at least. Throughout the course, emphasis is given in finding out weak points and suggesting how to fix them. This is usually done through chat sessions. As we solve each of your weak point, that can add a few more points to your score. Solve enough weak points and you may raise your score high enough to do really well. And who knows those few points can mean the difference between passing and failing, 98 or 99, or that dream residency or your second choice. ■

CHAPTER 3
EXPANDING YOUR LIMITED MEMORY

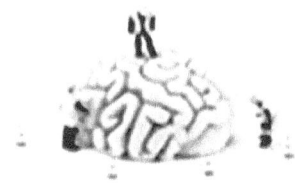

The question is, how do you go about expanding your limited memory. Technically, your memory capacity is relatively fixed. It's an innate trait. You are born with it and it's hard to expand it. But there are ways to make it more efficient so that you can store more information on the same memory space you have. We will discuss these individual methods in detail.

Organize the Information

One of the best ways to increase the amount of material you can cram into your limited memory is to organize the information you are studying into your head. This is one of the reasons why it is important to organize the information and not just study them at random. If you look at textbooks and reviewers, the information is organized by headings and subheadings. Taking the time to memorize this headings and subheadings initially can use up a lot of time. But over the course of your prep, you will realize that not only will it help you save time as you will find it easier to remember and recall more information later, it can help you do better in the exam by helping you to find the correct answer much more easily. We will discuss all the other ways organizing information will help you do better in the exam when we reach the section on how to study. At this point, we'll discuss how organizing the information will help you store more information that you can retain and recall quickly and efficiently.

To illustrate, imagine your memory as a table with only a few things on top. You can actually just throw those things on top any which way you want. It will not be hard to find a specific item you want. And any item that went missing you will know immediately. And adding a few more items on top will not be a problem.

On the other hand, imagine the same table and heaped on top of it is a pile of items 3 feet high. If it's not organized, it will be hard to find a specific item in that pile. You won't even know if any item is missing. Adding any new item to the pile will just make finding things even harder and there will come a point when the whole pile may just come tumbling down.

However, if you organize the items into groups, maybe create pigeonholes where each group of item can be placed, it becomes easier to find any item no matter how many items there are. It's just a case of knowing what group the items belong to. It's easier to know if any item is missing and when you have any new items to add just put them in the right group and you won't have problems finding it.

In practical terms, once you have the headings and subheadings memorized, any new information you encounter, just put them into the right classification, and relate them to the related information in your head. You will be able to remember and recall that information much better than if you just try to memorize that info as a single piece of fact. This is why it is best to study concepts in an organized fashion through the use of textbooks and reviewers. Studying concepts randomly as when most people use q banks as a study tool can make it harder to remember them.

Since I was a kid, I had always organized anything I learned and store them in my head that way. In fact during my Steps, whenever I cannot recall any information immediately, I will go through my memory, imagine the outline in my head and dig for the answer. In a lot of cases, I just need to see the cover of the book I used to organize the information in the first place and the answers will come out. We'll discuss this in more detail and practical applications of this principle under the section on how to study

Different Types of Recall

There are many ways we store information in memory and how we store them affects the way we recall them. It is important for us to recognize the different types of recall and how to make use of them in our prep.

There are actually 4 different types of recall, but not all of them are considered useful for the USMLE.

1. ***Immediate Recall*** - This is the most important type of recall when it comes to the USMLE. They are things you can recall immediately without any problem. It is so familiar to you that recall is instinctive. An example is your name. You don't really have to think about the answer.

2. ***Aided Recall*** - This type of recall is important in the USMLE primarily because of the limitations of immediate recall. They are things you can recall easily given time and some clue. It's called aided recall because you need some form of memory aid in order to recall the bulk of the information. Mnemonics are good example.

3. ***Familiar Recall*** - This type of recall usually forms the bulk of things we are able to remember. They are things you can recall given enough time and lots of clues. A good example is when you have read and studied something for the first time. The topic is very familiar to you but you have a hard time recalling all the details. This is also the case for things you used to know very well but some time have passed since you learned them.

4. ***Learnable Recall*** - These are things that you knew before but have already forgotten. This is usually due to the length of time since you have encountered these topics. It is easier to relearn them than to learn something you have not known before. That is why an old medical graduate can review for the USMLE but someone who has never studied medicine before, cannot just review for it without going to medical school first. Of course there are really brilliant people who are exceptions but this rule holds for most of us.

For the purpose of the USMLE, familiar and learnable recall are both too slow, i.e. takes too much time to recall and useless in a timed exam like the USMLE. Therefore only immediate and aided recall is important in the USMLE.

Immediate recall is very fast but also has a very limited capacity. In a timed exam like the USMLE, immediate recall is the most important type of recall. The larger your immediate recall, the more information you can retrieve very fast, the more questions you can answer in a given time. It would be good if we can put all the things we have studied in the USMLE into immediate recall, but due to its limited capacity, we cannot. So best is to put all the high yield stuff into immediate recall and as much low yield stuff as possible without displacing the high yield ones. The rest we put into aided recall.

Aided recall is much slower than immediate recall.

However, its capacity is several times larger than immediate recall. Due to the huge amount of information you need to learn and be able to recall for the USMLE, immediate recall is not enough and you need to use aided recall to store all the data. Its main disadvantage is that not only is it slower than immediate recall and therefore slow you down in a timed exam, you also need a clue that has to be stored in immediate recall. Although most people using mnemonics uses a nonsense keyword as a clue, personally, I do not advise it. Due to the limited capacity of immediate recall, it is preferable to use high yield information as your clue words rather than nonsense mnemonics. One way to do that is to use headings and subheadings as clues to aided recall. We'll discuss this in more detail in the section on How to Study.

The question of course is how do I put information in familiar recall to immediate recall and aided recall and aided recall to immediate recall. What about learnable recall, what do I do about that?

Well, for learnable recall, you relearn the material again. It will be much, much faster than learning it from scratch. Then it will now be in familiar recall. Things in familiar recall can be upgraded to aided and immediate recall using the 3 R's of retention and recall. We'll discuss the 3 R's in a while. Ditto for getting things in aided recall to immediate recall.

We stated that it is best to put high yield stuff in immediate recall and lower yield stuff in aided recall and that you make use of the 3 R's to do that. Therefore it is important to design your prep to make use of these facts. First by using two types of notes, one containing high yield material another containing both high yield and low yield material. Then design it so you spend more time on the high yield stuff than low yield stuff. In the course, the prep is designed to insure that you cover the right material in the right proportion so high yield stuff winds up in immediate recall more than low yield ones.

Key to Improving Retention and Recall

Making use of the 3 R's is the best way to improve retention and recall.

1. **Relation** - It's easier to memorize things that are related to what we already know. While children can memorize by rote, adults find it more difficult to memorize things that way. It's easier if they relate it to something they already know. Another thing to take note is that the more relationship or links that 1 piece of information you know has to other information, the stronger you are able to retain and recall that information. In fact information that is located in immediate recall has the most linkages with other information you know.

2. **Recency** - The more recently you have encountered a piece of information, the better you are able to remember it. As time passes, you tend to forget. This is both a blessing and a curse. It's a big disadvantage because of you don't encounter any piece of information regularly, it tends to fade. However, you can make use of this principle to remember specific things more strongly than others. For example, high yield stuff vs. low yield ones.

3. **Repetition** - The single best method to remember anything is by repetition. In fact, you can force yourself to remember anything by sheer repetition. The problem with repetition is that it is also the most time-consuming and for some people the most boring way to memorize anything. That is why it is best to use the principle of recency and relation to shorten the total amount of time you need to memorize something than through repetition alone.

The course is actually designed to insure that you make full use of the 3 R's to maximize your ability to retain and recall information. First, you need to do at least 3 revisions. Some of my students ask me if it means reading 3 times. The answer is it depends. If you can fulfil the goal of each revision by reading only once, then yes it means reading 3 times. But based on my experience very few people can meet the goal of each revision by reading only once. Some may need 2 or 3 readings just to meet the goal of one revision. Another frequent question is if I mean that you should revise Pathology 3x, then Pharmacology 3x, etc. No, I mean revise Pathology, then Pharmacology, etc. all seven subjects one revision, then go through all seven subjects again for the second revision, etc. This makes use of the principle of recency and repetition to cement your mastery of the subject.

Throughout the course, you are also asked to memorize headings and subheadings and relate details to them. You are also asked to do within subject integration and between subject integration as well. Lastly, at least for the big three, you are asked to complete a chapter quiz after each chapter and move on to the next chapter only if you achieve a minimum score. More importantly, if you fail to meet minimum score requirements, you are required to repeat reading through the whole chapter rather than just what you got wrong. Again it's a basic application of the 3 R's to strengthen your mastery of the subject. The reason you do per-chapter quiz only on the big three and not all 7 subjects is that doing per chapter quizzes and repeating whole chapters is very time-consuming. But due to the sheer importance of the Big Three for USMLE Step 1, it's worth the extra time to do it this way.

Make Information More Compact

If you look at textbooks vs. reviewers, you will note the same information can be presented in different forms. Long explanatory sentences with lots of discussions and examples like in textbooks, or short compact form in the form of bulleted lists, tables and illustrations like in reviewers. You can actually store more information in compact form than in long explanatory sentences. We will tackle the different methods we can do this under the section Right-sizing the USMLE. ∎

CHAPTER 4

RIGHT-SIZING THE USMLE: MAKING INFORMATION MORE COMPACT

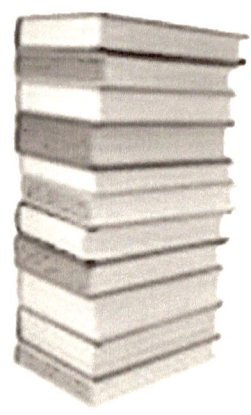

Because our memory capacity is limited and the amount of information we need to know for the USMLE is vast, we need to make information more compact so as to fit our limited memory capacity.

First, we need to understand that some topics are considered more important than others. We need to understand high yield topics vs. low yield topics.

Second, the level of detail you are expected to know about each topic varies. Therefore, it's important to study the topics in the right level of detail for the exam.

Third, different types of study materials present the topics at different levels of compactness. Therefore, using the right study material can impact the total number of topics you can actually squeeze into your limited memory.

Lastly, even though there are 7 subjects in Step 1, the emphasis given by the USMLE for each subject actually varies. Therefore, it is important to allocate the proportionate amount of effort to each subject in line with the emphasis given to it by the USMLE.

High Yield vs. Low Yield?

High yield topics are topics that have a very good chance of coming out in the exam. Low yield topics on the other hand are topics which come out less often. It is important to note that although high yield topics come out more often, it's never 100% of the time. Although low yield topics come out less often, it's never 0. In order to do well in the exam, you need to study both high yield and low yield topics but you need to master the high yield topics more.

One of the more common errors people do when studying for the USMLE is to do a high yield review only and depend on the online Q banks to cover the low yield stuff. The problem with studying this way is that we tend to remember more, topics we studied later and therefore reviewing this way, you tend to remember the low yield topics more than the high yield ones. One way to correct for this tendency is to do one more round of high yield review before the actual exam but after finishing q banks.

Worse of course are those who only cover high yield topics in their prep. Even if they are able to remember every high yield topic they study, they barely know enough topics to pass this exam. If they happen to remember only 90% of what they studied, they would fail.

Mastery, Know and Familiar

You do not need to study every topic in the same level of detail in order to do well in the exam. The level of detail that the USMLE expect you to know about each topic differs. We can classify the different level of detail into 3.

- Topics you need to **Master** are topics that USMLE require you to know in every detail. An example is HIV/AIDS. It presumes you know everything about it and the questions asked in the exam reflect the need to know the topic in detail.

- Topics you need to **Know** are topics that the USMLE expect you to know in detail, but it does not have to be at the level of detail as the topics you need to master. A good example is Pancreatic Neoplasms.

- Topics you can just be **Familiar** with are usually low yield topics or topics that are of interest only to specialists. A good example is the different types of transcription factors. Questions that require you to just be familiar with them will usually give you enough detail in the question stem itself.

Different Types of Study Materials

Although you need to study and understand a lot of topics in the USMLE, you do not need to memorize all of them. You only need to retain and recall the more important topics and in varying level of detail.

When you start your revision for the USMLE, the first step is to read and understand the concepts tested. The best study materials to use at this stage are textbooks and lectures. Textbooks are usually long, with detailed explanations and lots of examples. They presume that you know next to nothing about the subject at hand. Lectures meanwhile, cover topic highlights that you need to pay special attention, too. But come time to memorize, retain and recall the materials, textbooks and lectures are too bulky to be memorized and retained. We all know this instinctively, that is why we always take down notes from the texts we read and lectures we listen too.

After reading and understanding the concepts, we need to memorize, retain and recall those concepts. The best way to do this is to memorize those same information in compact form or what we call notes. This is usually in the form of bulleted lists, tables and illustrations. There should actually be two types of notes when you are studying for the USMLE and the main reason is that you need to memorize both high yield and low yield stuff and knowing which are high yield vs. which are low yield helps you study more efficiently.

Study Notes are notes that cover everything that will come out in the exam including both high yield materials and low yield ones. They differ from textbooks in that they are presented in the form of bulleted lists, tables and illustrations, rather than long explanations and examples. They cover most of the information covered in textbooks but in more compact form with shorter explanations and limited examples. They also exclude materials not covered in the USMLE. An example is Kaplan Lecture Notes and my Pathology Study Notes.

Outline notes are even more compact than study notes. It's just bulleted lists, tables and illustrations with no explanations at all. A lot of the texts are telegraphic with some composed only of a word and a phrase. They contain only high yield stuff and rarely anything else. A good example is BRS and my Pathology Outline notes.

Memorizing textbooks wastes time and limited memory space. Plus it takes more time to recall the same information. Memorizing and retaining more compact information in notes is more efficient and conserves both time and memory capacity which are very limited. And it's faster to remember and recall an illustration than explanatory text.

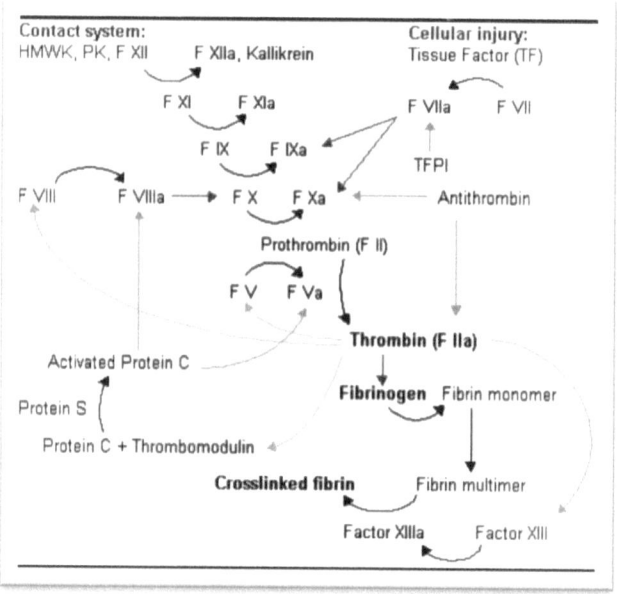

For example, the coagulation cascade can be memorized using a one page illustration. That same illustration can be as long as 5 pages of explanatory text in a textbook. Memorizing a one page illustration is faster and uses less memory than 5 pages of text. Recalling the same information is also much faster if done this way. However, if you have never studied or do not understand the coagulation cascade, you will need those 5 pages of text to understand the one page illustration. But once you have studied and understood the concept, memorizing the details using that one page illustration is easier.

Although notes can be used for improving recall, it's better used for studying and memorizing information. Both flashcards and q banks are the most effective way to improve recall. The best types of flashcards are those that contain only one piece of information per card. The problem with most commercial flashcard is that they contain too many information per card. For example on a typical microbiology flashcard, you have the name of the micro-organism on one side and all the details on the other side all on one card. That makes it harder to practice recall using those kinds of cards. The main reason commercial flashcards are written that way is to make it easier to memorize the information for each topic. However, if we understand that notes are the best way to memorize information, we are better off using notes for memorization and flashcards for recall.

Q banks on the other hand are very effective for improving recall. They are also effective in teaching you the finer points about different topics. They can be used to highlight what you thought you know or understood but did not. They can also be used to teach you how to use what you know to think through problems and how to solve them. Therefore, Q banks are an essential part of your prep if you want to do well in the USMLE.

Different Emphasis given on Different Subject by the USMLE

Not all the subjects covered by the USMLE are treated with equal importance in the examination. Just as some topics are more important than others, some subjects are given more weight by the USMLE.

The approximate weight given by the USMLE for each of the seven subjects in Step 1 is as follows:

- *Pathology and Pathophysiology ~ 40%*

- *Pharmacology ~ 10% - 15%*

- *Microbiology and Immunology ~ 10% - 15%*

- *Anatomy ~ 8% - 10%*

- *Physiology ~ 8% - 10%*

- *Biochemistry ~ 8% - 10%*

- *Behavioral Sciences ~ 10% - 12%*

As you can see, the biggest weight given by the USMLE is Pathology. This means almost half the questions you will encounter in the USMLE are questions on Pathology and Pathophysiology. This is followed by Pharmacology and Microbiology and Immunology which range from 10 - 15% of the questions you will encounter in Step 1. Together, these 3 subjects account for 65% of all the questions you will find in the exam. Together we call them the big three. It is important to spend most of our prep on these three subjects as they account for the bulk of Step 1.

This does not mean however that we can ignore the other 4 subjects or what we call the minor 4. They still cover ~ 35% of the exam and can significantly impact your score. Behavioral Science occupies the biggest percentage of the minor 4. However, almost half of behavioral sciences are medical law and ethics. And these are best learned using cases through the online Q bank. Anatomy contains a lot of facts that needs to be memorized, while physiology and biochemistry contains lots of concepts and process that needs to be understood and memorized. However, in Step 1, you will find most of the questions in Anatomy, Physiology and Biochemistry integrated into the Big 3. This is due to the clinical slant of the USMLE. Therefore, the best way to study for Step 1 is to concentrate on the big 3 and integrate the smaller subjects into them.

If you go through the forums or even other prep courses, they usually start by asking you to take a quiz to evaluate which subjects you are weak in, then to study and improve your score in that subject. That is probably a very good idea if the USMLE treats all the subjects with equal weight. But we know that is not the case and so long as you are weak in the big three especially pathology (below 70% in q banks for passing, below 80% for scoring high) then you should concentrate on the big three even if you are scoring below 50% in the minor 4. Your overall performance will improve faster that way.

The best way to study for Step 1 is to allocate the appropriate amount of study time and memory space commensurate to the weight given to each subject by the USMLE. It is both more efficient and more effective in helping you get a good score. ■

CHAPTER 5
MINIMIZING THE FORGETTING PROCESS

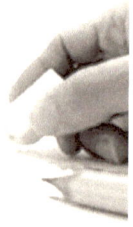

Do at least 3 Revisions

The best way to minimize the effects of the forgetting process is to do at least 3 revisions. This is not the only reason for doing 3 revisions however.

People have always asked me if doing 3 revisions means doing 3 readings. The answer depends on the person. Each revision has a purpose. And if you could achieve that purpose with one reading per revision than it's technically 3 readings. But if it takes you 2, 3 or even 4 readings for each revision to achieve the goals, then so be it.

So, what are the goals of each revision?

1. First Revision - Memorize the concepts for each subject and integrate those concepts within the same subject

2. Second Revision - continue memorizing concepts but also integrate concepts between subjects

3. Third Revision - master the concepts and fill in any gaps in your knowledge

Retain Enough Information with Each Revision		
	Percentage remembered	Length of Review
Before First Revision	20%	
After First Revision	80%	3 months
Before Second Revision	40%	
After Second Revision	85%	1.5 months
Before Third Revision	68%	
After Third Revision	92%	3 weeks

During first revision, you need to memorize and be able to recall the concepts for each subject. If it takes more than one reading to achieve this then do so. It is also important to integrate topics within a subject. For example in pathology, topics in General Pathology should be integrated in Systems Pathology. General Pathology discusses pathologic processes that are common across different organ systems and tissues. For example, cell pathology, inflammation, immune reactions, neoplasia, etc. However, the actual Pathologic processes that occur in the different organ systems do differ in some cases and these differences are discussed in more detail in Systems Pathology under each organ system. A good example is cell death under cell pathology. Cell necrosis is generally the same with all cells, but there are characteristics specific to each organ system, eg. coagulation necrosis in the heart vs. liquefactive necrosis in the CNS.

Other examples include integrating Basic Bacteriology to Clinical Bacteriology. Basic Bacteriology discusses general features of bacteria, like cell walls, life cycle, etc. You need to understand these general characteristics, link them to how these characteristics differ in the individual bacteria which is discussed in Clinical Bacteriology. It's important to study this way as a lot of questions will test your understanding of these general characteristics and how they relate to individual differences in specific organisms. Same thing holds true between basic virology and clinical virology.

During second revision, you concentrate on integrating topics between subjects. It is important for us to understand that medicine as a whole is a very large concept. It's very hard to learn such large concepts at one go. So we break it up to smaller concepts called subjects. It's easier to learn these concepts in smaller chunks like anatomy, physiology, pathology, etc. In fact we divide them into even smaller concepts, for example, cell pathology or even into systems like CNS, cardio, etc. However, studying per subject, per system limits our knowledge of these concepts. Therefore, there is a need to integrate these concepts so we know medicine as a whole and not in parts. Since our patients are whole persons, we need to treat them as a whole and not in parts, so only by knowing medicine as a whole can we be effective physicians.

Knowing the parts and not being able to see the whole limits our understanding. It's like the story of the 7 blind men and the elephant. Since they are blind, they can only use their hands. So the blind man holding the trunk insists the elephant is like a snake. The one holding the ear insists that the first man is wrong and that the elephant is more like a large carpet. The one holding the legs insists that they are both wrong because the elephant is like a large column. The 4th man insists that an elephant is a wall as he tries to push on the elephant's body. Therefore integrating all the different topics and subject together is important in understanding medicine and the USMLE tests whether you understand how everything fits together or not. That is an important difference between the USMLE and the shelf exam which is per subject.

We will discuss in more detail how to integrate between subjects when we talk about how to study.

The third revision builds on the first and second revision. You continue to memorize the concepts and integrate and memorize the integrated topics. At this stage, you also concentrate on identifying your weak points and cover them. That is the reason why you start online q banks at this point.

You may be wondering why you still have weak points. If you followed the course for your first two revisions, then you have actually covered everything in your prep, so why will you still have weak points? The main reason is that everyone has things that interest them more than others. If you are more interested in one thing you pay more attention to it. If you are not interested in something, then even if you are reading it, your mind may not be wholly in it. You may zone out while going through that particular topic or wander to something that interests you more. So by the end of your prep, even if you covered everything in your review, you will be stronger in some things more than others.

However, the USMLE does not really care what topics interest you or not. If it's important, it will show up in the exam. Therefore, you need to be strong on topics that will come out in the exam whether you find it interesting or not. So you need to cover your weak points.

Practice Good Retention and Recall Techniques with each revision

It is important for you to maximize your retention and recall of what you have studied in each revision. You need to practice the 3 R's of retention and recall every time. Relate any information you encounter to information you already know. Then make sure you repeat what you have studied as often as needed for you to retain what you have read. The best way is to repeat it out loud. As if you are talking to someone. For more complicated concepts, I try to explain it out loud either to someone or to myself. Or draw out the process in a piece of paper or whiteboard. This helps me retain the information well. Using flashcards are also very helpful in improving recall.

Insure you have retained enough information in each revision

Throughout the course, you are told evaluate your progress even during the first revision. For the big three, you do per-chapter quizzes for the first revision and per-subject quiz on the second revision. For the minor 4, you do per-subject quiz on the first and second revision. The reason for doing this is to insure you have retained enough information and be able to recall them before moving on to the next chapter. This will insure that not everything is gone from your head by the time you are taking the next revision.

To illustrate: For example, before you start your first revision of chapter 1 of Pathology, you remember 20% of the topics discussed from medical school days. After revising, you have retained 80% of the topics in the chapter and you tested this using the recommended per chapter quiz. Of the 80% of the topics you have forgotten you are able to absorb 75% of what you don't know or a total of 60%. 20% + 60% = 80%. However, it took you 3 months to finish your revision, so by the time you start your 2nd revision, you have forgotten half of what you know and you are down to 40%. You do your second revision and you remember 75% of what you have forgotten. That's 45% out of 60% so 45% + 40% = 85%. So you now retain 85% of the topics for the chapter. However, it took you 6 weeks to finish your 2nd revision. It's faster than the first revision because you still remember a lot of what you had studied in the first. They are mostly in familiar recall and aided recall, so easier to retain. The shorter review means you forget less so you retain 80% after 6 weeks which is 68% out of the 85% you originally retained. When you start your 3rd revision, you recall 68% of the topics discussed in chapter 1 of Pathology and you are able to retain 75% of the 32% you have forgotten which is 24%. so after third revision you recall 92% (68% + 24%) of the topics discussed in chapter 1 of pathology.

As you can see, it is important to make sure you retain enough information at each revision to insure that your retention and ability to recall the materials you have studied will steadily improve with each revision. The only way to make sure of this is to test for it as you finish each chapter. If you do not set a minimum score you want to achieve in each revision, you will wind up not knowing enough to pass the exam even after 3 revisions.

To illustrate, if you achieve only a score of 40% after revision 1, you might hit 50% at revision 2 and 55% at revision 3 which is still a failing score. Therefore, revising without testing how much you have retained and able to recall at each step of your revision can result in a very poor outcome.

You might be wondering why you don't sit for the exam immediately after you finish your third revision when your retention of the material and your ability to recall the same is at its peak. If the USMLE is the kind of exam that only requires you to be able to recall what you have learned, then that is your best strategy. However, just being able to recall what you have learned is not enough to do well in the USMLE. You need to be able to use what you have learned to analyze cases presented. You need to be able to answer difficult questions that would otherwise be easy to answer if presented in a different manner; you need to be able to do this under time pressure in an exhaustive and taxing environment. So just being able to recall what you have studied is necessary but does not guarantee you will do well in this exam. You need to be able to do more than that.

Finish Your Prep in as Short a Time as you are able

We know that as time passes, we tend to forget things. This is called our rate of forgetting and the rate is a function of time, in other words it is constant. Therefore to keep forgetting to a minimum, we need to make our prep as fast possible without sacrificing quality. It is useless to finish your prep fast but wind up retaining less to nothing. It is important to make sure that you are prepping properly and using your time wisely. Prep fast but prep right. ■

CHAPTER 6
STRETCHING YOUR LIMITED TIME

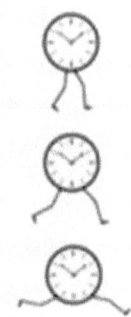

Study Longer on a Daily Basis

You will do a lot more progress studying continuously for 7 hours in one day than stretching the same 7 hours over a week by studying one hour every day for 7 days. The main reason for this is that it takes time before we reach our peak studying time, i.e. what I call the *'zone'*, where your concentration is at its peak and your ability to absorb and memorize information is most efficient. Usually, when we start reviewing, it takes time for this peak to happen. For me it's about 15 to 20 minutes. So if you study only 1 hour a day, you are at peak for only 40 minutes per hour or 280 minutes for those 7 hours. If you study 7 hours in one day, then you will be in peak form for 400 minutes for those same 7 hours, resulting in more progress.

Another reason why this is true is that your rate of forgetting is constant. You forget a little of what you have studied every day and it stands to reason that you will forget more in 7 days than in 1 day. By studying huge chunks per day, you limit the amount of forgetting you do.

Review Continuously, Avoid Long Breaks

A very common mistake that I often see especially among Old IMG's is that they fail to review continuously. They will review for a few weeks, and then take a few weeks break because they have to take care of something then come back to restart their review. Then they wonder why they are making very slow progress. In fact, some people do these breaks often enough or long enough that after months of prepping they are right back where they started. The main reason why this is a problem is that our rate of forgetting is constant, while our rate of learning is variable and depends on a lot of factors.

In fact, given two people who are equal in intelligence, study skills and other abilities and studied exactly the same things, in the same level of detail, the person who finishes his prep in 3 months will have retained and be able to recall more material, then the person who took six months to finish his prep. Therefore it is very important that you avoid long breaks during your prep and try to finish it as fast as possible without sacrificing the quality of your prep. On the other hand, don't go thru it so fast that you wind up retaining nothing because you are just too intent on finishing x number of chapters in x number of days.

Always Get a Good Night's Rest

Studies have shown that it is when we are fast asleep that memory is transferred from short term memory to long term memory. Therefore, it is important to get enough hours of sleep every day, so what you study everyday actually gets stored in long term memory and not gone in a few days.

In medical school, a lot of us are used to cramming late at night for a quiz or exam and it works since you can usually retain information in your short term memory for a day or two. But you will notice that information you gained from cramming is gone from your head in a few days, while things you memorized systematically over days with adequate sleep you will tend to remember longer.

Since cramming seems to work in medical school, a lot of examinees make the mistake of cramming for the USMLE and in most cases with few exceptions, realize too late that cramming does not work for the USMLE.

Take one day off a week and do anything but study

It is a known fact that we are only human, and we all have the tendency to burn out. Prepping for the USMLE is a very long process and therefore there is a real need to pace yourself. Many people make the mistake of studying too hard to the point of exhaustion. Thus they burn our before completing their review. You need to take one day off a week. And during your day off, you do anything but study. Take that day off to recharge your batteries. Trying to plough on when your mind is exhausted results in no real progress and is just a waste of time. If you work during the week, studying at night and can study for a full day only on weekends, then take Friday evening offs. To make sure you are fresh and well-rested during the weekend when you do the bulk of your prepping.

Keep your attention focused; take breaks between long periods of review

So you have decided to review for 8 to 10 hours per day. It is actually not a good idea to review continuously for 8 to 10 hours straight without short breaks in between. Your concentration will wane, your mind will start to wander and your progress slow down. It is best to have breaks between periods of study. What the optimum ratio between study time and break time differ from individual to individual.

In my own case, I work best with a study time of 1 hour and 40 minutes with a 20 minute break. It may be different for you. I suggest you first try studying 45 to 50 minutes and take 10 to 15 minute breaks in between. Then adjust according to what works best for you. It does not have to be exactly 45 minutes, just more or less. If you are in the middle of the chapter and your break time comes, try to finish it before taking the break. If you still have five minutes and you just finished one chapter and you know you can not finish the next chapter in that time, then break there.

If you really can't stand not studying anything for break, then you can change pace by doing some flashcard review or do speedbuilding exercises in answering question. How to use flashcards and how to do speedbuilding exercises will be discussed in more detail later.

Foster a good learning environment

The best way to insure that you maximize your prep time is to foster a good learning environment. What exactly is a good learning environment? Well, it's slightly different for different people, but in general it's an environment that allows you to concentrate and stay focused in your review to maximize learning. It's an environment that keeps you relaxed and comfortable and not tense or tiring. It is an environment which is free from day to day worries that distracts you from learning. Even though for most of us it's impossible not to be distracted by day to day problems, it is important to create this ideal learning environment even only for a few hours each day, to allow progress in your studies.

Some may prefer to study in libraries, but for me libraries are too distracting especially with lots of people around. Even if they are quiet, I find myself people watching all the time.

And then the occasional loud whispers can break my concentration. Others may prefer a garden environment, sitting under a tree or a park bench. For myself, I prefer my own room. I study best when I can move from sitting down to lying in bed to pacing around depending on the mood of the moment. I prefer to explain aloud concepts I am trying to understand and master and talking to myself in public tend to make me self-conscious.

It is understandable though why some prefer to study outside their home. Noisy children, uncooperative roommates and party-going friends can make it hard to study at home. If you have children, then make sure you get somebody to babysit for you as it is impossible to look after children and study properly at the same time.

If you have to work for a living then make sure you are financially prepared for reviewing. In my case, I was a practicing physician, six months before starting my prep, I was saving money and my social life went to zero. For the first 5 and a half months, I worked part-time while prepping and for the last 6 weeks, I took a leave from work, endorsed my patients to my colleagues and concentrated on prepping. That was only possible because I was financially prepared for it. Too many times, financial problems or even disasters have derailed study plans and schedules or even caused people to give up taking the exam. ■

CHAPTER 7

MAXIMIZING YOUR SCORE:

GETTING THE HIGHEST SCORE YOU CAN

Different people have different expectations when it comes to how they think they will do in the USMLE. These can range from just passing the exam to getting high 99's. For the past 7 years that I've been in the forums, writing my blog and teaching hundreds how to pass this exam, I have noticed that a lot of people fail to match their expectations to their abilities. I have seen people who are good enough to get 99's just expecting to pass and not exerting enough effort commensurate to their ability. I've also seen people who have no chance of getting 99's burning themselves out trying to achieve something beyond their capability.

I have learned that it's really very hard to accurately gauge how you will perform at the beginning of your prep. Only after prepping for some time, noting your progress and how effective your studying is going can you decide how well you can perform and whether a 99 is achievable. In my case, as a very old IMG, at the beginning I thought, 85 would be good. Then halfway through my prep, I realize that I could easily get a 90 or a 95. It wasn't until the last few weeks before the exam, when I was going through the online q banks did It dawn on me that 99 was a huge possibility, so I went for it. Only after I did my NBME evaluation exam did I realize I could get a high 99 and did.

Therefore, the best goal to aim for is to try to get the maximum score you are able. If that happens to be a 99, well and good, if not, at least you know you did your best and got the best score you can get. Personally, I believe a lot of people who passed this exam could have gotten a much higher score if only they tried harder.

Factors that affect your performance

Memory Capacity

Your memory capacity is an innate trait and will severely limit the total amount of information you can store at any one time in your head. This is one of the most important factors that will affect how high your score can go. It is a general rule that all things being equal, the more information you have stored in your head and are able to recall, the higher your score will be. Although, there are various methods to improve the efficiency of your memory capacity, there are limits to how much improvement you can actually make.

Analytical Ability

Most questions in the Step 1 require some analysis to be able to answer correctly. However, a significant number of questions require very good analytical skills to answer. Inability to analyze fast or well can severely limit the score you will be able to get.

Although Analytical ability can be trained, it usually takes a long time to do so; therefore we can consider analytical ability to be a relatively fixed ability. Usually analytical ability is trained during college years where you are taught how to think through. Things like logical reasoning and critical thinking. If by the time you have finished medical school and you still are very weak in this area, then it would be hard to improve on this much during the short time you have for USMLE prep.

However, given enough time, even people with poor analytical skills can figure out most things eventually and if you have poor analytical skills, you need to make use of this fact to improve your actual performance in the exam. One of the reasons it's hard to do on the spot analysis to answer questions in the USMLE is the severe time constraint imposed on each question. So you tend to run out of time before you can finish analyzing the question and come out with an answer.

Therefore, you need to make your analysis before the exam. If you have done the analysis before the exam, then during the exam you will not be spending time analyzing, just recalling the result of your analysis. There is a systematic method of figuring out the most probable way questions will be asked and what information needs to be analyzed in the exam. For example, Goljan's Rapid Review and his live lectures have done a lot of analysis on the topics covered, so you only need to memorize the results of the analysis and don't need to do the analysis yourself at the time of the exam. That reduces the time you need to answer that question. That's one of the reasons that listening to his lectures can significantly increase your scores. We will discuss later how to anticipate what questions will come out in the exam and what topics you need analyze before the exam.

How well you studied

This is actually the only factor that you can do something about during the limited time you have for prepping. That is why it is important for you to know how to prep properly for this exam. You really have only one chance to do well in this exam. If you pass this exam with a score of 75, then that is your score and you cannot retake the exam. If you fail the exam, although technically you are allowed to take it up to 7 times in some states, for most residency program, failing this exam even once can close the door to that program for you or make it very hard for you to get in.

Therefore, it is important to prep properly from the start: To study effectively and efficiently. To correct bad study habits. To remedy each weak point in your prep so you can get the highest score you are able. Throughout this course, we will identify your weak points and help you find a remedy for the situation.

Factors that affect your learning speed

Intelligence

Intelligence determines how fast you understand and learn concepts. The higher your intelligence, the faster you learn period. Intelligence is an innate trait and training can increase it very little. Therefore, if your intelligence is low, then you will have a hard time learning the materials for this exam. However, it is estimated that in order to finish medical school in the four years allotted for it and perform adequately, you need an IQ of at least 120. So if you did finish medical school, we know that to a certain extent you are above average in intelligence.

Ability to absorb information

The speed with which you absorb information is also a very important factor in learning speed. Some people are very good at memorizing, retaining and recalling information more than others. Intelligence is a factor in your ability to absorb information, but not the only one. The ability to remain focused and concentrate is also important. There are lots of intelligent people whose ability to retain and recall information is less than stellar. And not all people who are intelligent have photographic memory and vice versa. Again there are ways to improve this ability but only to a limited degree. The potential is mostly innate and therefore hard to change.

How fast you forget

Your rate of forgetting affects your learning speed. Your learning speed is a function of your rate of learning minus your rate of forgetting. Some people tend to forget things faster than others. This affects the total amount of things the person can retain after studying. This also means that this person tends to go into plateau early. It is imperative that if your rate of forgetting is fast you need to keep a tight schedule and stick to it. Any delay could prove fatal for your review.

Reading speed

How fast you read has a very big impact on your review. The faster you are able to read, the faster you are able to go through the materials you have to study. If you have poor reading speed, this could impact your prep a lot. Being able to read fast also helps you later when you start answering questions. The less time you spend reading the question proper, the more time you have to spend recalling, analyzing and answering the questions. Later, we will discuss the various ways you can increase your reading speed. Although technically you can double, triple and maybe quadruple your reading speed. That will take probably take years of practice. In the few months you spend for your prep, the most you can hope to achieve is to increase your reading speed by 20 to 50%.

Environment

One of the most important things you need to have in order to enhance your learning speed is to have a good learning environment. Study in an environment that will allow you to concentrate and focus on your review with litte or no distraction. If it involves removing yourself from your normal day to day environment then do so. If you can't create a good learning environment, then be prepared to take a longer time to be prepared for this exam.

Plateau and Decline

So long as your rate of learning is faster than your rate of forgetting, your performance will continue to improve. However, there comes a time when your rate of learning declines. There are various reasons why this happens. The most common reason is that you have filled up your memory capacity and it gets harder to cram in more information. Sometimes, it is due to the fact that you are burning out. This is usually due to taking too long to prep. However, as we said before your rate of forgetting is always constant. when the point comes where your rate of learning is equal to your rate of forgetting, your scores stop improving and you have reached what we call the plateau and further studying won't raise your scores.

Eventually, there will come a point when your rate of learning becomes slower than your rate of forgetting. At this stage you go into decline and delaying the exam further to study will lower your score even more. To avoid this you need to monitor your progress as your exam date nears and watch out for plateauing, which is indicated by a lack of progress despite continuous reviewing.

The key to maximizing your score

In the end, everybody plateaus. Some will plateau with a 95, some with an 85. Others will plateau at a 99. That is true for everyone. What you hope will not happen is that you plateau with a failing score. The key to maximizing your score is really to time your exam date to when you plateau. Earlier, you are still improving and those extra points are wasted. Later and you run the risk of going into decline. Of course if you plateau at a failing score, you should not take the exam. The usual cause for plateauing at a low score is due to poor study skills leading to poor prep or taking too long to study which can lead to you burning out before you have studied enough to get a good score.

In my experience with myself and the hundreds of students who have gone thru my course, most students plateau at between 6 to 8 months. The shortest is about 3 months and the longest about a year. If you do plateau at a failing score or a score way below what you want, your option is to take a break, anywhere from 2 weeks to 2 months should suffice and redo the complete prep. If you are following my course program, that means doing all 3 revisions a second time around. You should be able to go thru the revisions faster this time as a big percentage of what you have learned and memorized are still there. Two of my students have successfully done it this way. One went from failing to a 91. Another went from a predicted score of 80 to a 99. So it's doable.

If you plateau at a failing score because of bad study habits, then taking a break and redoing your review may not help you much. You need a whole new study program to improve your performance. It has never failed to surprise me when I see people who have failed to pass this exam multiple times continue to prep on their own and using the same study program and study skills to boot. If a person is dying of a disease which you have repeatedly tried to cure yourself and failed. Do you continue to try to cure it yourself, or is it time to ask for help? Same with prepping for the USMLE. ■

* * *

unit 2

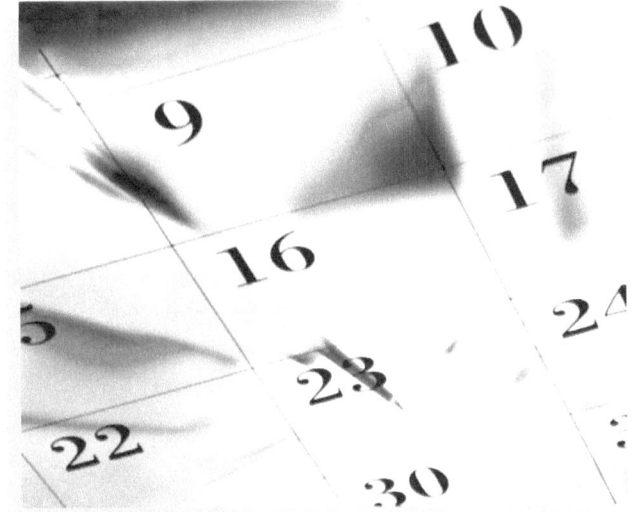

Scheduling Your Prep

CHAPTER 8

INTRODUCTION

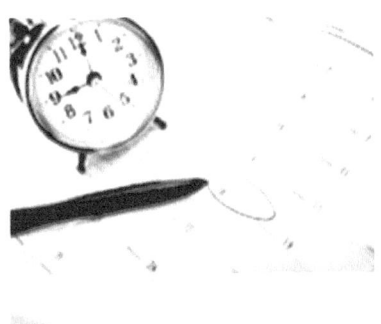

A few years ago, I went through a forum and read a post that went like this. *'Hi Everyone, I'm new here. I'm an IMG and I graduated 8 years ago. I am scheduled to take Step 1 in 5 months. What do I do now? Please help.'* I remember thinking that this guy is in very deep trouble and I would not want to be in his shoes. These shows how unprepared he was for this exam. Before you even sign up for the exam, you need to know how you would tackle this exam, how long a prep time you would probably need to insure you would at least pass or better yet get a good score.

If you go through the forums, you will be surprised at how many people would jump into this exam without knowing what they are getting into. They think that going through First Aid a few times and wham, they're ready to pass what is probably the toughest medical board exam in the world. Worse, some even expect to get a 99 as if by magic. If it's that easy then how come the failing rate for IMG is 40%. Of course, the stupid explanation is that 40% of all physicians in the world are too stupid to pass Step 1, which is patently ridiculous. To understand why US medical students perform better in the USMLE, please read these posts in my blog.

Importance of Proper Scheduling

The best way to insure that you prep properly and that you are able to cover everything you need to study so that you will pass and maybe even do well, is to create a proper schedule for your prep. It requires you to consider your present capability and circumstances, how much time you need to achieve a level of competence to pass this exam and if you are desirous of getting a high score, how much additional time you need to do what is needed to achieve the desired score. Therefore to properly schedule your prep you need to know your capacity to learn, what your current situation is and what results you want to achieve. Only then can you create a schedule that will increase your chance of achieving that score.

Why you need 3 phases in USMLE Review

It is important for us to understand that studying for the USMLE is multi-dimensional. First you need to understand the topics covered by the exam. Then you need to memorize them, that is, to be able to retain and recall them in the right level of detail for the exam. Lastly, you need to be able to recall them in the context required by the USMLE, under time pressure, with difficult questions that require analysis to be able to answer correctly. In summary, you need to learn, to memorize or master the topics, then learn how to answer USMLE type questions. To accomplish each of these tasks require different skill sets and different study materials, so it's best to divide your prep into three phases which we will discuss in more detail later. You need to take these three phases into consideration when you schedule your prep.

Briefly, the 3 phases are as follows,

- *Learning Phase* - You need to understand concepts before you can even start memorizing them. You cannot master what you have not learned. The only people who can completely skip the Learning phase are incoming third year medical students. And even then for some of them, it may be a good idea to do it anyway.

- *Mastery Phase* - Just understanding concepts is not enough if you want to do well for this exam. You need to be able to retain and recall the concepts at the right level of detail. And you need to be able to do very fast and under time pressure. Therefore, you need to master the topics not just know them.

- *Test Preparation Phase* - Any exam is supposed to test your knowledge alone, but in practical terms, it is impossible to isolate the effects of the modality used from the results of the exam itself. Therefore, the type of exam and its mechanics in the end will have a huge effect on the end result. The test preparation phase is where you train to get used to answering USMLE type questions and minimize the effects of the mechanics of the exam itself on your score. The more you are able to minimize its effect, the better your actual score approximate what you truly know.

Why you need to create a study plan

Actually the process of creating a study plan is more important than having a study plan. The propensity of people to borrow or follow another person's study plan fails to amaze me. And surprisingly, these same people seem to believe that the same study plan will work for them just as well as it did for someone else. Nothing is farther from the truth. Although general principles on how to prep do exist, they serve as guide only and the best study plan are those created for your particular situation. Unless your friend is your clone and you have similar strengths and weakness and your life situation is the same, it is likely that any study plan which works for him will not work for you.

We will discuss how to create a study plan for the USMLE Step 1 in more detail later. What is important is before you can create a study plan, you need to evaluate your circumstances first. Then you need to understand your study skills and capabilities so you can estimate how fast you learn and absorb material. Then you need to properly estimate just how large USMLE Step 1 is so you do not underestimate the amount of learning you need to do. Only then can you make a realistic study plan that will apply to you.

Why use a schedule organizer

Be aware that no matter how carefully you plan your prep schedule, it is inevitable that surprises and crisis will spring up once in a while, given the length of time involved in prepping for the USMLE. Therefore, any schedule you create for your prep should not be written in stone. It should be a living document that adjusts to the circumstances you find yourself in. A good schedule organizer will show you everything you need to do for your prep, your target date of completion for each task, & your actual performance in relation to each target date. Any adjustment you made to the schedule in light of your actual performance should be noted on the organizer.■

CHAPTER 9

THREE PHASES OF USMLE REVIEW

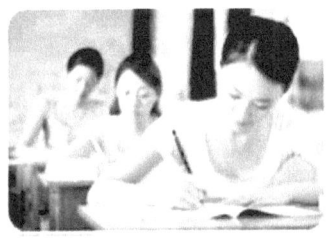

It is important for us to understand that the USMLE is a very complex exam. Studying is a very complex activity that requires various skills in order to do well. And yet for most people, studying for the USMLE involves just reading books or maybe listening to lectures. Although these activities do contribute over all to studying for the USMLE, there are a lot of other activities you should be doing if you really want to do well on the boards.

The activities involved in learning a topic is bit different from those needed to memorize and retain them in great detail. The activities involved in becoming proficient in a type of exam and mechanics of an exam is also different from the first two. We call the first two phases, the *learning phase* and the *mastery phase*. The third one is the test preparation phase. This is true for any exam.

However for short exams, we usually do them at the same

time and sometimes skip the test preparation phase. For longer exams, we occasionally separate the first two phases and may or may not do a test preparation phase, i.e. do practice questions. But for really long exams, where it is crucial to score well, like the USMLE, it is best to separate all three phases as you will get the most improvement in results that way, and also make it easier to pinpoint where you botched your review and focus corrective action.

Each phase requires different skills, activities and study materials. Therefore it makes sense to organize the activities and study them in order.

Learning Phase

You cannot review what you do not know. You cannot master what you have not studied. Therefore, the first step of your prep should be to make sure you know all the concepts to be tested in the USMLE. This is usually done during the learning phase. There are various approaches to the learning phase but the basic principles are the same.

First, your main purpose is to read to understand the medical topics that will be tested on the board. You should not try to memorize them in detail at this stage. Reading to understand requires detailed explanations and lots of example. Reading to understand may also require you to go through the topic multiple times in order to make sense of what is being discussed. The best materials to use at this stage are textbooks and lectures.

Second, understand, you sometimes need to know certain concepts first before you can understand other concepts. Basic concepts build up to more advanced concepts. For example, it is very hard to understand Pathology unless you understand Anatomy and Physiology. So if you are studying a concept in Pathology and find it hard to understand, it may make sense to study the anatomy, physiology and biochemistry related to that concept. Basic concepts in Pharmacology come from Physiology and Biochemistry so you need to understand them first before Pharmacology can make sense.

Third, you may need to go back to materials you have read before in order to integrate the various medical concepts together. For example it is best to start with Anatomy, then Physiology. You then integrate Anatomy and Physiology, correlating structure and function. The next step is to study Biochemistry and integrate it into concepts in Anatomy and Physiology, e.g. Cell Biology and Physiology, etc. When you read Pathology, you need to integrate them into Anatomy, Physiology and Biochemistry.

We will discuss in more detail how to study for the Learning Phase under the section on *How to Study*.

Mastery Phase

For the USMLE, it is not enough for you to know and understand the medical concepts tested in the exam. In order to do well, you need to master the concepts in the right level of detail for the exam. Mastering involves memorizing, retaining and being able to recall concepts tested in the exam at the right level of detail and at the speed required by the USMLE, which is usually around 1 minute for each question.

You need at least 3 revisions in order to cover everything you need to do during the Mastery Phase. Memorizing and retaining information is never easy, especially if you need to retain large amounts of them like in the USMLE. You need to do at least 3 revisions in order to do well in Step 1. In general, the more revisions you do the higher the score you will get but only up to a point. Therefore do at least 3 revisions, but be prepared to do more if you want a good score.

You need to memorize the concepts at the right level of detail for the exams. A lot of times, the main reason people do poorly in these exams is they fail to memorize the concepts at the right level of detail for the exam. If you go to the forum, most people complain that all the questions look familiar and they feel that they know the concepts being tested, but they keep on coming up with the wrong answer. The main reason is that you need to know a certain level of detail about a concept before you can answer the question.

For example, the question gives you 5 clues in the stem for you to answer the question. You need only 3 clues to answer the question but due to the lack of detail in your knowledge, you only recognize two of the clues. You will fail to answer the question. Another example, you have 5 clues in the question stem and you recognize all of them. However, this time the question is more difficult and require you to know two additional details that you do not know and are not in the stem that you need to relate to the question stem in order to come up with the answer. Again you are unable to answer this question.

So what level of detail should you study for the USMLE Step 1? Actually that is a judgment call, and the better the judgment call, i.e. the more you are able to study medical concepts tested at the level of detail expected by the USMLE, the better your score. Throughout the course, I have tried to make sure we cover everything at the right level of detail expected by the USMLE.

You need to be able to recall concepts in a timely manner not just memorize them. Another mistake that a lot of people who are prepping for the USMLE make are to assume that once they have memorized the concepts, that is enough. But the USMLE imposes a tough standard that you should be able to recall what you know very fast, usually in a minute or less or it presumes you do not know it. You don't even get partial points.

For example, a lot of times in the middle of the exam, you can't recall a piece of information needed to answer the question. You think you must have forgotten it. However, a few minutes after leaving the exam room, the answer comes tumbling out. It means you have not really forgotten it and that given enough time you can recall it. But this is the USMLE and if you cannot recall it, you don't know it. Therefore, you need to practice recall not just memorize and that is done during Mastery Phase and well into Test Preparation Phase.

Problems in the Learning Phase can impact it. You cannot master what you do not know; you cannot review what you have not studied. If you do not understand the concepts you are trying to memorize, you will have a hard time doing so. Therefore, you need to do the Learning Phase properly. Minor problems in the learning phase can usually be resolved by just going back to textbooks as you encounter them during Mastery Phase. But any major problem and you may need to go through a formal Learning Phase.

Test Preparation Phase

Most people's Test Preparation Phase is composed of doing online q banks and that's it. Actually, there are a lot of things you can do in your Test Preparation Phase to help you raise your scores significantly. Taking the time to do your Test Preparation Phase properly is worth the time and effort if you want to do well in the USMLE.

The main purpose of the Test Preparation Phase is to learn how to take USMLE type examination. Although the purpose of any examination is to test your knowledge of the concepts being tested, in reality, the type of exam you are taking and its mechanics greatly affect the score you will get in the end. Therefore, you need to be so used to the way the USMLE exam is conducted that the mechanics, methodology, testing environment, etc. stop becoming a significant factor in your final score and your score will reflect as close as possible to what you really know.

First, you need to know how to answer USMLE type questions. Although the USMLE questions are probably some of the best constructed questions ever, it does follow a certain pattern and therefore knowing these patterns can help you perform better in the examination.

For example, most of the questions are primarily multiple choice questions or MCQ. Training to answer MCQ question is slightly different from answering an essay type question or enumeration question. In MCQ, the correct answer is always one of the choices; therefore you always have a chance of getting the correct answer so long as you don't leave anything blank. In an essay type question, so long as you get most information into your answer you get points. In MCQ, it may ask for a specific detail that you don't know, so even if you know most of the concept being tested, unless you know the particular detail of the concept being tested, you don't even get partial points.

The USMLE also has certain methods of making an otherwise easy question tougher. Knowing how this is done and being able to deconstruct a tough question to an easier one can help tremendously in getting to the right answer much faster. We will discuss these in more detail later.

Next, you need to correct bad habits in test-taking. With the choice of using MCQ for standardized tests, bad habits in test-taking have arisen which most test makers exploit in order to make the exam harder. Due to the fact that in MCQ, the correct answer is always in the choice, most test takers have gotten used to looking for the answer among the choices. In other type of exams like enumeration, fill in the blanks, essay, etc. you need to have the answer in your head immediately after reading the question since there is no list of answers to look for it.

The USMLE exploit this bad habit by putting in distractors or require two-to-three step thinking to be able to find the answers. Distractors are answers that are very close to the right answer that unless you are very sure of the correct answer, you may chose the distractors rather than the correct one. It may be based on a common misconception prevalent in society but medically wrong, an age-old medical concept that has just been proven wrong or radically revised, or medical concepts that are the same in all aspect except in one small detail and you need to know that detail to answer the question correctly.

Questions requiring two to three step thinking are questions in which the answers in the choices are not immediately related to the question concerned. You need to relate the answers to a fact not mentioned in the question stem, nor in the choices in order to be able to find the correct answer. Three step thinking questions require you to link an unnamed fact to another unnamed fact in order to get the right answer. For example, the question presents a medical case but does not tell you the diagnosis. The question instead of asking what the diagnosis is asked instead the major side effect of the treatment of choice for this case. You first have to be able to diagnose the case, then you need to know the treatment of choice for this case, then you need to know the most common side effect. If you are unable to connect the chain of facts, you won't be able to answer the question.

You need to get used to the USMLE CBT interface. The USMLE exam uses a computer based interface that does unfortunately takes time and practice to get used to. You need to get used to navigating through the various screens. Otherwise, you waste valuable time during the actual exam figuring out the interface. And since this is the USMLE, time is always in short supply. There are a lot of features in the interface, which you may find useful or not. And you need to test how useful they are for you before you even sit for the exam.

For example, the normal findings for laboratory examinations are available in tabular format through the CBT. However, it does take time to open the tables, look for the tests and find the normal values. Therefore it may make sense to memorize the normal values for the more common laboratory so you minimize the amount of time navigating through the tables looking for them. Plus it may be worth your time to be familiar with which tables a particular laboratory finding may be found so that you can go directly to the right table. Another thing I did was when I went to look for a normal value on a table; I write it on the writing board provided by *Prometric* so I don't have to search through the tables again in case I need the same normal values again.

You need to get used to time-pressured 7 hour examination. People think that all they need is to study the topics to be tested, do some q banks and they are ready to tackle the USMLE. That is akin to someone who thinks since they can run two km in the track; they should have no problem running a 24-K marathon. They just need to run the 2K but do it 12 times. The marathon is a whole different animal and so is the USMLE. The time pressure and length of the exam will take its toll on your performance and if you lack the stamina to last the eight hours (including 1 hour break), you can fail. You also need to know how to time your breaks. You will be surprised how quickly time passes in the actual exam. Just signing in and signing out when you take a break can take almost 3 minutes. So you need to be ready for it.

Do you need to do all three Phases?

In order to do well in the USMLE, you need to make sure you have covered all three phases properly. However, depending on your current situation, you may not need to go through all three phases. For example, if you just finished your first 2 years of medicine in a US medical school in most cases, you can skip learning phase and proceed to Mastery and Test Preparation Phase directly. If your school provided you with prep sessions, you can even skip most of Mastery Phase and just go to high yield review and then Test Preparation Phase. (i.e. First AID and online q bank. If you are an IMG (including Caribbean students) who just finished your first two years, some of you may be able to skip learning phase. It depends on how good your medical school is and how well your own performance is. For most IMG, however, you may need a formal Learning Phase. If you are an old IMG, then Learning Phase may be crucial to your success, as most likely your knowledge is somewhat obsolete or you have forgotten most of what you have learned. However if you have done some prep before, you may be able to proceed without a formal Learning Phase even if you are an old IMG. ■

CHAPTER 10
HOW TO CREATE A STUDY PLAN

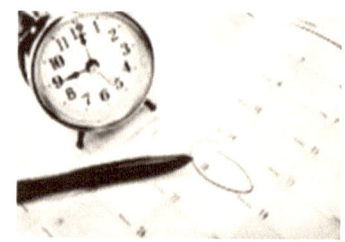

Why Create a Study Plan

This is probably the question foremost in the mind of anyone who ever thought of tackling the USMLE. I remember when I was starting out, how this pre-occupied me a lot. Although studying for the USMLE is a big endeavour, studying how to study for the USMLE is no mean feat either. Just like an architect or engineer needs to plan out how to build a building before actually building it, we need to plan out how to prepare for the USMLE before we even begin studying.

Now some people can just jump right into reviewing and 3 to 5 months later take the exam and come out with a 99. I'm not one of those and so are, I believe, majority of those taking the USMLE. Some will start by applying and scheduling an exam 5 months later, only to find out that they're not ready. So they extend their period of eligibility and still they're not ready. Some will take the exam and fail or score so low that it amounts to the same thing. Some will forfeit the application fees and reapply later. Of those who do, some wind up getting good scores because they've learned their lesson and did better preparation this time, while for others the results are going to be poor because they did not change anything they've done before. Proper planning is crucial for proper preparation

Steps to Creating a Study Plan

Often, in forums, I've heard people refer to taking the USMLE in military terms. Going to War against the USMLE, they call it. Military generals never go to war without a thorough battle plan, that is if they expect to win and neither should you. We'll be tackling this topic head on.

The Steps to creating a study plan are:

1. Determine your objective

2. Know thy enemy

3. Know the learning process

4. Know the components of a good study plan

5. Know the factors that can affect your study plan

6. Scheduling

7. Importance of sleep, rest and recreation

8. Putting it all together

Determine Your Objective

Just like all battle plans, you start out with what is your main objective.

1. *Is it to pass the exam?*

2. *Get an average score?*

3. *Beat the mean?*

4. *Ace it?*

High scores isn't everything in the match. But it can make up for other deficiencies in your resume, like less than stellar grades in medical school, older grad, lack of USCE, etc. Often you see people in forums posting their study plans and asking if it is enough, but enough for what? Determining your objective is the first step in assessing whether your study plan is adequate or not.

So how high a score should you aim for? Well, it is a universal truth that most people do not achieve what they aim for so it is a good maxim to aim high. In the Greatest Salesman in the World, Og Mandino stated that

"It is better to aim for the moon and hit an eagle then to aim for the eagle and hit a rock."

If you aim for a 75 and fail to reach it, you are in trouble. If you really want a 99 aim for a high 99 so you have points to spare in case not everything went as planned.

One word about setting objectives is to never set it in stone. As you finish your study plan and even as you begin your studies, you may find that your objective may change. Either you've underestimated yourself and have found out that you could do better, or your situation's change, (e.g. your wife gets pregnant or you got pregnant, lost your job, got promoted, etc.) Do not be afraid to reset your objective; just be aware how it will impact your overall chance in the match.

We've often heard about how people downgrade their objectives when they are unable to follow through on their plans. But how often have you heard of people who failed to upgrade their objectives when presented with the opportunity.

In 1863, on the first day of the Battle of Gettysburg, when Gen. Robert E. Lee's Confederate Army defeated the Union Soldiers defending the three ridges south of Gettysburg, Lt. Gen. Robert Ewell refused to take Cemetery Hill, which wasn't part of the original Battle Plan, even though it was lightly defended at that time. On days 2 and 3 after Cemetery Hill was reinforced by Union troops, the Confederates made numerous charges to take Cemetery Hill to no avail. This led to the famous Pickett's charge by 12,500 Confederate troops on the 3rd day of battle which was repulsed by union rifle and artillery fire at great loss to the Confederates. By refusing to upgrade his objective, Gen. Ewell missed an opportunity that could have changed the outcome of the war and the destiny of the United States.

Know Thy Enemy

Now like all good Generals, we have decided on our main objective for the USMLE. The next step is to study the nature of the enemy, only then can we know how to defeat it.

Now someone might say, why don't you just post a study plan and like good soldiers we will follow them. Well that would be easier for me, but I doubt it will work or be effective for a lot of you. You see, a plan presumes that there is an objective, takes into account where you are coming from, your skills and particular strengths and weaknesses and your particular condition. A one-size fits all plan presumes you have the same objective, the same skill sets, the same background and the same prevailing environment which is just not true.

Now normally when somebody asks you how to go to Times Square, you presume he is somewhere in NY. But in the internet, the person may be in San Francisco, Baltimore, London, Karachi or even Manila. And the answer would be different in each case.

So too must your study plan be different depending on your particular circumstances. Just as a doctor tailor makes his treatment plans depending on your circumstances (*child, adult, geriatrics or healthy, immunocompromised, debilitated*) we must tailor make our study plans accordingly. But just as doctors have treatment guidelines to guide them in formulating a good treatment plan, so too does this book attempt to provide you with guidelines on how to study to help you formulate a good study plan.

The purpose of the USMLE Step 1 is to test your knowledge of Basic Science concepts relevant to the practice of Medicine and to that extent it has been faithful. All questions you will find are related to the basic sciences like pathology, microbiology, pharmacology, etc. However, to emphasize its relation to the practice of Medicine, a lot of the questions are in the form of clinical vignettes. In Step 1, most of the Clinical Vignettes are classical presentations rather than atypical presentations.

Another thing you'll notice is that whereas in Step 2 and 3, the cases are usually common diseases, Step 1 cases include a lot of diseases that are fairly uncommon. The reason is that USMLE Step 1 emphasizes basic sciences and sometimes, important basic science concepts are illustrated by uncommon diseases. For example, *Angelman and Prader-Willi Syndromes* are fairly uncommon but demonstrate the principle of Imprinting. Small cell CA of the lung demonstrates the concept of para-neoplastic syndrome but is actually less common than squamous cell CA or AdenoCA. So this should guide what you should emphasize on your review.

All USMLE Steps also require you to be able to recall all this information in a minute or so. What you cannot recall, you do not know as far as the USMLE is concerned. So knowing something is not enough, you must be able to recall it too. Increasingly, questions are 2 to 3 step in order to avoid aided recall from the answer choices themselves.

All this impacts what we have to study, how we study and what steps will be involved in our review in order to be able to do well in the exam. We will talk about how we learn and master information and how to apply this in coming up with a study plan for the USMLE.

Know the Learning Process

We now have our objective and we know what the USMLE wants us to know and in what form it will test us for that knowledge. The third part is to understand how we learn and accumulate knowledge.

I've found the following to be a useful framework for analysing and understanding where I am in my review and assess my strength and weaknesses. Using this framework will help us not only in preparing our study plan, but also in assessing any problems we have during our review and remedying them. We can divide our review preparations into 3 parts.

Knowledge Acquisition (KA) - This is where you put information into your Knowledge Bank (KB) Most new graduates are extremely fine here (Except if you're one of those who barely made it. Crammed for every test and promptly forgot everything afterwards. Most Old graduates and some IMG graduates usually have problems here. This can impact how long your review period should be and the amount of "hitting the books" you have to do.

Knowledge Recall or Review (KR) - This is how well you extract information from your KB. Most new graduates have some problem only here. FA and the Q Banks make a fantastic tool for improving Recall. So people with problems here (New grads mostly) usually give fantastic ratings to FA and Q bank. Other methods to improve recall include flashcards and group discussions. If you have a KA problem, you still have to do KR after you have remedied your KA problems.

Test Preparedness (TP) - If you are not familiar with CBT, MCQ or clinical slant to questions, this is where your problem is. Problems with sitting for 8 hour exam are also classified here. Difficulty in answering 2 to 3- step-thinking questions and running out of time during the exam also falls here. This is where Q Banks are the most effective.

How long, how detailed and how demanding your study plan will depend on where you are standing right now. If you have lots of KA's to do, then you have your work cut out for you. Textbooks may even be in order and not just Study Notes and Outline Notes. If it's mostly KR, then repetition,

repetition and more repetition is the way to go, especially outline notes and Q banks. If it's TP then Kaplan and UW Q bank will be most helpful.

Know the Components of a Good Study Plan

We now discuss the different phases of a complete study plan. The three phases are as follows

Learning Phase: This is where you try to learn everything that you still do not know about medical concepts tested in the USMLE. You need to do KA here to fill up your KB.

Mastery Phase: at this point, you already know the concepts, you just need to put them into immediate recall so that you can recall them in the minute or so that USMLE requires. This is mostly KR with some KA.

Test and Psychological Preparation: It is important to prepare yourself both physically and mentally for the gruelling 7 to 8 hour exam *(16 hours for step 3)*. Failure to do so may mean low scores or worse failing the exam altogether. It is also at this point that you improve your test-taking ability and get used to taking USMLE type exam.

Many people tend to skip the learning phase and go directly to the mastery phase by purchasing review books like FA or BRS then use them almost exclusively for their studies. Depending on your goals and your current situation, this could be either a minor problem or a catastrophic one. One cannot master what one does not know. You can't review materials you do not know. You need to study them.

The longer you are out of medical school the more time you need to spend here. The lower your scores were during medical school, the more you need to concentrate in learning all the important concepts tested by the USMLE.

Even recent graduates who are very good students cannot remember everything they've studied and usually there are gaps in their knowledge due to a variety of reasons. (E.g. Subject not covered by professor, etc.) Therefore, it still makes sense to realize that there will be concepts you do not know and the best place to prepare for them is during the learning phase. This is especially crucial because you should not schedule your exam before you finish your learning phase (a common mistake committed by many). You should only schedule the exam once you are in your mastery phase where the time frame for accomplishing most preparations is more predictable. We will deal with scheduling later.

The mastery phase is what most thinks of when they talk of reviewing and in truth for most people; this is where most of their preparations should be. The main objective of the mastery phase is to get as many information as possible into immediate recall so that one can do well in a timed exam like the USMLE. Given enough time, one can recall almost anything one has learned and that's the reason USMLE is a timed exam. It wants to test how much material you've mastered rather than how much you've learned. Outline notes, Qbanks and Flashcards are the way to go during mastery phase.

The test and psychological preparation phase is also very important but most often the psychological preparation phase is commonly skipped and yet many times this can be crucial to doing well in the examination or even passing it. Even if you are physically able to finish 8 hours, being mentally alert by the 6th to 7th hour is not that easy. Horror stories abound of people panicking and going blank during the examination. Even the test preparation part commonly involves only doing online q banks when there are a lot more things you can do to increase your chances of doing well.

In boxing for example, Boxers do not do much training in the last week before the fight. They've finished their training by then and if they've not, then there is a big chance they will lose. However, they still go to the gym not to train but to keep focus and to prepare themselves for the upcoming bout. Therefore, it is important to give yourself time before the exam to physically recuperate from a long and arduous preparation and mentally focus on the upcoming examination.

Know the Factors That Can Affect Your Study Plan

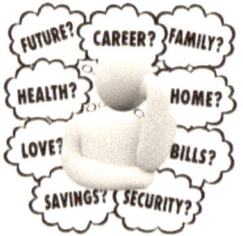

We will now discuss the various aspects that make making a one size fits all study plans practically impossible. This will be just an overview and we will discuss them in more detail later.

An important factor that will affect how you prepare for the USMLE is your background.

- *Are you a recent graduate or an old one?*

- *AMG? Or IMG?*

- *Good student acing all exams? Or barely made it through medical school?*

- *Top school, run of the mill or diploma mill?*

- *English as medium of instruction or other language?*

- *Native English speaker or poor in English? (Having to translate the questions in your head can just be enough to break the exam for you.)*

Any of these factors will affect how you prepare, how long you prepare and what additional steps you have to take in order to be ready for the USMLE.

Another important factor is your strengths and weaknesses and particular skill sets which you possess.

- *Fast reader vs. slow reader?*

- *Good comprehension skills vs. weak comprehension skills.*

- *Good memory and retention vs. poor memory and retention.*

- *High IQ vs. very High IQ. (It is presumed that since you finished medical school, you probably have a high IQ or at least above average. A minimum IQ of 125 is needed in order to reasonably finish Medical school in the time allotted for it.)*

- *Whether you study better by reading, listening to lectures or group discussion.*

- *Long attention span vs. short attention span.*

- *Good concentration vs. easily distracted.*

- *Strong self-discipline vs. poor self-discipline.*

- *Favorite subject. (You tend to learn and retain better information on subjects you like and if they happen to be heavily tested subjects, i.e. Patho, Micro and Pharma in Step 1 or IM in step 2 and 3, this could influence how well your review will go. If you hate them, it will be harder.)*

Last, but not least, your present circumstances can affect not only your study schedule but how high a score you should be aiming for.

- *Working full time, part time, jobless.*

- *Head of the Family and sole breadwinner*

- *Pregnant*

- *Have small kids particularly toddlers and infants*

- *Amount of Social support you can draw on*

- *Parents take care of all financial needs (The social pressures from relatives can be particularly demanding in this situation.)*

- *Family expectations*

- *Visa issues*

- *Your age and your health*

All of the above circumstances will affect your study plan. It will also affect your schedule including when you should schedule your examination. Let's look at them in more detail.

Your Educational Background

We will discuss how your educational background affects your study plans. We will go to the different aspect of your background.

New grad vs. Old grad

High scores are more important to an old grad. Also the need for longer study time and additional responsibilities like work and taking care of kids makes their study plans much more complex and demanding than for new grads.

AMG vs. IMG

IMGs need higher scores and longer study schedules than AMGs. AMGs have an advantage in Behavioral Sciences. US medical schools prepare AMGs to do well in the USMLE. This includes special pathophysiology classes and clinical correlations. While most IMGs are left on their own to integrate the concepts, it's the reason for the popularity of Goljan's lectures. When he goes "mechanisms, mechanisms, mechanisms", he means "pathophysiology, pathophysiology, and pathophysiology."

To read more about the alleged differences between the difficulty of the exam for AMGs and IMGs, refer to my blog post "Is the version of the USMLE for IMGs harder than for AMGs?"

Good Student vs. Barely Made It

If you barely made it through med school, then there probably are large gaps in your knowledge of concepts tested by the USMLE. It is important for you to hit the books, especially on frequently tested concepts you have not mastered. Even if you were a good student, there could still be some gap in your knowledge and it pays to go through outline notes like FA or BRS to find weak points.

How to Master the USMLE Step 1

Top school, run of the mill, or diploma mill?

There are topnotch graduates from diploma mill schools and there are really bad students from top schools, but on average you expect students from top schools to do better, therefore your school can affect how much preparation you need to make.

English as medium of instruction

Even if you are proficient in English, having learned medicine in a foreign language can affect you. Most medical terms are not taught or learned outside of school. English is the medium of instruction at our school. Although I am proficient in both Filipino and Chinese, I learned medical terms in Filipino only after long practice and still have difficulty with medical terminology in Chinese.

Native English Speaker or Poor in English

The USMLE is in English and having to translate medical terms and even regular words in your head can slow you down a lot. In a timed exam like the USMLE, it could prove fatal. So if you have language problems, work on it first before attempting the USMLE.

Your educational background can and will impact your performance in the USMLE. Make sure you take that into consideration in your preparation.

Your Strengths and Weaknesses

We will deal with how your particular strengths and weakness impacts your study plan. Different people possess different skill sets. Your particular skill set will determine how you should conduct your review.

Fast vs. Slow Reader

Fast readers have a tremendous advantage in reviewing. If you are a slow reader, read up on some tips to increase reading speed in my blog. Also fast readers have an advantage when tackling the kilometric questions that appear in Step 2 CK.

Good Comprehension Skills vs. Poor Comprehension Skills

If you have poor comprehension skills, compensate by rereading the topics if needed. You need to understand it to learn it. What matters if you finish fast but did not learn anything? Again, main reason why you should not schedule examination until you finish your learning phase, since how fast you learn is variable.

Good Memory vs. Poor Memory

Memorization is just repetition. If you have poor memory, do more repetition. Mnemonics is unreliable most of the time due to time constraints of the exam. Frequently tested material must be in immediate recall. Use mnemonics for more peripheral, less tested information. How to improve your memory is tackled in more detail in other sections.

High IQ vs. Very High IQ

If you finish med school then you can pass the USMLE. You just need proper preparation. The USMLE is tough but definitely doable. Having a Very High IQ just makes it easier.

Study Mode: Reading, Lectures, Group Discussions, etc.

Some people learn better reading, others hearing lectures and others by group discussion. As I said before people learn best by association. A lot of times you remember facts not because you read them, but because the lecturer said something humorous or you remember a particular incident during group discussions. Different people learn better in different environment. Understand what environment suits you best and include that in your study plan.

Good Concentration vs. Easily Distracted

Some people can study with the TV on while wearing an iPod and with children wailing in the background. Others need absolute quiet to study. You should determine under what environment you can study well. Phone calls, social events and other distractions will affect how long your preparation will eventually be.

Long Attention Span vs. Short Attention Span

Some can study for hours, while others get bored after some time. Schedule your review to take this into consideration. Short attention span can be offset by variety, either in topics reviewed or in study mode. For example, studying pathology and anatomy or physiology in parallel or alternately can offset boredom. Alternating between reading, taking short quizzes, group discussion and listening to lectures can also offset boredom.

Strong Self-Discipline vs. Poor Self-Discipline

Some people can make a study plan and stick to it. Others, well, others make a study plan and try to stick to it. *(wink..wink..)* If you lack self-discipline, it's best to recruit others to help you. Enrolling in a class (and showing up) can help. Joining a study group can also help. Do not schedule your exam in the hope it will force you to stick to the plan. You'll wind up losing $$ or failing the exam.

Favorite Subject

Pathology, Anatomy and Physiology are my favorite basic science subjects in Med School ---which just means that I tend to study and retain what I study on these subjects. You probably mastered more medical concepts in your favorite subjects than others. When reviewing for the USMLE you need to concentrate on the big subjects rather than what is your favorite subject. The big three is pathology, pharmacology and microbiology. If these are not your favorite subject then you know you have your work cut out with you. If they happen to be, then you probably can make do with less study time.

Your Present Circumstances

Each one of us has a life outside of studying for the USMLE. We will analyze how your present circumstances affect your study plan.

Working Full Time, Part Time, Jobless

Some people have to work full-time, which just means that they have to consider that their review period will be longer and that their schedule will be constantly interrupted. It is important for them to make sure that they set aside time for study and during those set time to isolate themselves from worries at work. The same could be said of those who work part time although their problem is not as bad as full-timer.

Head of the Family and Sole Breadwinner

Being head of the family and sole breadwinner is more challenging than just being employed. The pressure is physical, emotional and psychological. Having adequate social support is crucial if you want to pass or do well in the USMLE

Pregnant

Pregnancy brings with it a lot of problems not the least of which is going into labor at an inconvenient time (e.g. Like in the middle of the exam). Preparation for the exam and the exam itself are extremely high stress situation, so proceed with caution.

Have Small Kids Particularly Toddlers and Infants

Children are fascinating, cute and lovable except when they won't eat, become cranky and irritable. Then they're nearly impossible. Hats off to all USMLE takers who have toddlers and infants and still able to study well! For others, well, asking for help from other adult family members may be needed. So it is important to anticipate and prepare for this before start of preparation.

Amount of Social Support You can Draw On

Support from family, relatives and friends can make a

difference in your psychological preparedness for both the preparation phase and actual examination. There is a difference if people are rooting for your success or your failure.

Parents Take Care of All Financial Needs

Most new grads belong in this category. It is both a blessing and for some also a burden. The pressure to succeed at your first try because somebody else is paying for it can be overwhelming. Although for some there may also be a tendency to take it easy since they don't have to worry about the financial burden.

Family Expectations

High family expectations can be a spur to do well, or can hamper performance. Low family expectations can result in the same things as well. Again the result differs depends on each individual's particular situation and their reaction to them.

Visa Issues

You need to take the Step 2 CS exam in the United States and if you need a visa to enter the US, you will need to anticipate the time delay it takes to get one. So schedule your review with that in mind.

Your Age and Your Health

Suffice to say, younger people have more stamina than those older, although you can also say that older people may be wiser. In addition, poor health can affect concentration and study time.

Scheduling

Now we talk about scheduling. There are different aspects of scheduling that we have to consider. Foremost is in what order do I take the USMLE. For AMGs the answer is moot and academic, since this is dictated more by the medical school than personal preference. For IMGs, who are free to choose their own sequence, it is more problematic. While it is true that for some IMGs it is more beneficial to take the USMLE Step 2 CK, I believe that for majority of exam takers, taking it in sequence provides tremendous benefits. Please read my post on *which exam to take first* in my blog.

The next consideration is how long a preparation time should I allot for review. Again, this is so dependent on individual differences; it is hard to give an estimate. However, for the ideal graduate, meaning fresh grad, good student from good school, 2 to 3 months for Step 1 and 1 to 2 months for Step 2 CK is about average to pass and do well but not to ace the exam. (Again, there are geniuses who probably will be able to ace the exam, though) But outside of ideal, you will have to make adjustments.

Often, I see in forums people who will declare that they've signed up to take the examination in 5 or 6 months (or 2 or 3 or whatever), then ask plaintively, "what do I do now?" All I could do is shake my head since they are headed for disaster.

I have already discussed about the learning phase and mastery phase in your study plan. Mastery phase is most predictable. Usually 2 to 3 months to pass Step 1 on average and 3 to 4 months to ace it. Other factors like reading speed, IQ, available study time, etc. will affect it but the estimates are average. The learning phase is most unpredictable. That is why you should not schedule your examination until you are starting your mastery phase.

The last advice I can give is to schedule your exam to achieve a certain score rather than to finish by a certain date. By all means schedule your exam to finish by a certain date but if by that date you are not ready then postpone the exam. It takes as much time, effort and money to retake an exam as to cancel it and take it later. Except if you fail and retake it, it can do irreparable harm to your ability to match.

Importance of Sleep, Rest and Recreation

Having enough sleep, rest and recreation is very important

in the review process. The worst time to burn out is just before the actual exam day. Also, studies have shown that neural connections are made during sleep and that unless we sleep; whatever we have learned during the day is not stored in long term memory. Infants sleep all day, because they have more information to process than adults. So not sleeping to study is not considered good quid pro quo.

Rest breaks are also important within the day as monotony will tend to dull your attention. Your eyes may be moving through the words but your brain is not recording it. 45 to 50 minutes study with 10 to 15 minute break is a good rule of thumb although again, personal differences may mean you have to adjust the actual rest break.

Now, there will be people whose total review period will go beyond 5 to 6 months due to circumstances not within their control and as such, they will need to have a break. Burn out is a big possibility and it is better to extend total preparation time by a month to rest in between. ■

CHAPTER 11
SCHEDULE ORGANIZER

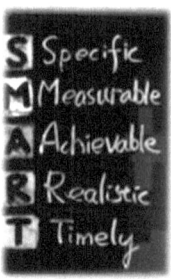

How to Create a Schedule

So, now you have planned out your prep. Created a viable study plan and put together a schedule for review. It is important to put all of this down on paper. Now a simple schedule just tries to arrange tasks and match them to the dates you hope to accomplish each of them. We'll use the suggested schedule for Askdoc's USMLE Prep Course for Step 1 as an example. Your actual schedule may vary depending on your study plan.

1. Learning Phase - 4 months

2. Mastery Phase - 4.5 months

3. Test Preparation Phase - 1 month

Since Learning Phase usually involves reading texts, you estimate how long it takes for you to read through all the texts. Usually it's best to learn them in the same order as you encounter them in medical school. You should also be aware that you need to integrate concepts in between your studying.

1.   Anatomy - 2 weeks

2.   Physiology - 1.5 weeks

3.   Biochemistry - 1.5 weeks

4.   Pathology - 5 weeks

5.   Pharmacology - 3 weeks

6.   Microbiology/Immunology - 2 weeks

7.   Behavioral Science - 1 week

Once you have finished your Learning Phase, you need to schedule your Mastery Phase. You need to schedule for 3 revisions altogether.

1.   First Revision - 12 weeks

2.   Second Revision - 4 weeks

3.   Third Revision - 2 weeks

Please take note that in the course the Third Revision is incorporated with the Test Preparation Phase. The 1st Revision for the minor three, namely Anatomy, Physiology and Biochemistry is incorporated with the 2nd Revision of Pathology and Pharmacology.

Schedule of First Revision is as follows:

1.   Pathology - 5 weeks

2.   Pharmacology - 2 weeks

3.   Microbiology/Immunology - 2 weeks

4.   Anatomy - 8 days

5.   Physiology - 5 days

6.   Biochemistry - 5 days

7.   Behavioral Sciences - 3 days

Schedule for the Second Revision is as follows:

1. Pathology - 10 days
2. Pharmacology - 6 days
3. Microbiology/Immunology - 5 days
4. Anatomy - 2 days
5. Physiology - 2 days
6. Biochemistry - 2 days
7. Behavioral Sciences - 1 day

Schedule for the Third Revision is as follows:

1. Pathology - 5 days
2. Pharmacology - 3 days
3. Microbiology/Immunology - 2 days
4. Anatomy - 1 day
5. Physiology - 1 day
6. Biochemistry - 1 day
7. Behavioral Sciences - 1 day

Using the Schedule Organizer

A static schedule will usually suffice for most people. However, for some people, it may make sense to use a schedule organizer. The reason for using a schedule organizer is that in a long prep process like what you undergo through the USMLE, you cannot plan for every contingency and schedule for it. Emergencies and other concern can crop into your schedule and you wind up having to adjust the original schedule to something that resembles reality more.

So how do you create a schedule through the schedule organizer?

1. *It must cover everything you need to do, so you can see what has been accomplished and what has yet to be done.* You need to know every chapter of every subject and make sure there's a spot for it in your schedule organizer. By doing this you will be able to see at any time what you have done and what you still have to do. People tend to underestimate the time they need to accomplish their task and the schedule organizer will help you see at a glance if your expected progress matches your actual progress.

2. *It must set good and realistic boundaries so you have enough time to cover what you need to do to accomplish your set goals.* You would be surprised at how many people set unrealistic time goals for their prep and wind up getting discouraged at their 'slow' progress. Understand that your initial schedule is based on a guesstimate. Therefore you need to be flexible. You can test your presumptions by noting how fast you are progressing and adjusting your final schedule accordingly. For example, you initially set 1 week to finish 5 chapters of Pathology. However it took you actually two weeks to do so, you now know that you will need to double your estimated time to finish your prep or you need to change your study methods so you can go faster or both.

3. *It must be flexible enough to cover for unforeseen circumstances.* Prepping for the USMLE is a very long process and it is unavoidable that things can happen that will disrupt your original schedule. You must be ready for it -which is part of the reason why you do not schedule an exam date until you have started your test preparation phase and you are meeting goals both in terms of time and performance. By this time you would have a more accurate assessment of when you can finish your prep and be ready for the exam.

4. ***It must be reviewed weekly and changes done as needed.*** You need to keep your schedule alive and update it regularly to reflect your current realities and circumstances. In order for your study schedule to effectively help you plan and map out your progress, you need to update it regularly, preferably once a week. Do not be like lots of people who make their schedule when they start their review and never look at it again. A few months later, they wonder why they have made so little progress.

There are a few things you need to consider when you create your schedule

1. Remember you need to do at least 3 revisions. Therefore, the prep process is long although each revision does get faster to finish as you redo them.

2. You have a limited time to finish your prep. You cannot study forever. There comes a time when you have to stop studying and sit for the exam. Or you have to stop studying because you have burned out. A flexible schedule is important, but too much flexibility can result in procrastination, i.e. the inability to finish your prep.

3. You need to accomplish a lot so as to pass the exam and even more if you want to ace it. Just passing this exam requires a lot of work and you have a limited time to do it. Acing this exam requires even more work and the question is do you have the time to do all those studying. You need around 10 x the amount of effort to get from 95 to 99 as to get from 85 to 90. Effort is not additive but exponential.

4. Efficiency in review means you try to keep to schedule and at the same time try to do everything you need to do to achieve your goal. You should try to keep to schedule and still achieve your desired goal. However, if you are unable to do so, you either have to extend

your period of review or lower your goal. My suggestion is you do a little of both in order to insure you do sit for the exam in the end. I remember a student who vowed he wanted a 99. Since it was not really possible for him to achieve this score, he kept on extending his prep schedule that in the end, he failed to sit for the exam at all. ■

***

unit 3

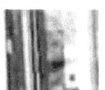

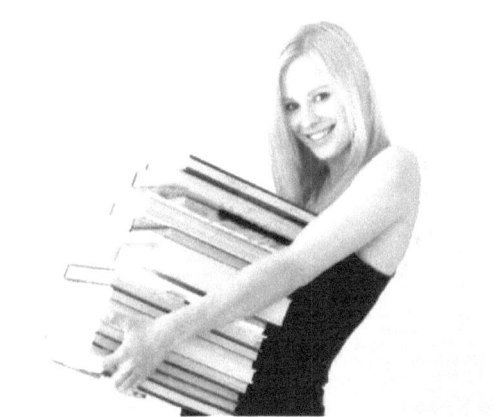

How to Study

CHAPTER 12

INTRODUCTION ON HOW TO STUDY

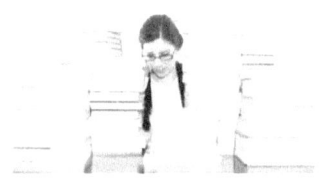

Why you need to know How to Study?

One of the most common question people ask me is 'Why do I have to learn how to study? I already know how to study, else how did I pass medical school?' It is true that as we go through the educational system we do pick up some skills in studying, but the amount of skills varies with each individual. And believe me, most people have relatively poor study skills compared to the top 10% of students.

The amount of study skills you need in order to do well in an exam rise in proportion to the difficulty and complexity of the exam. And the USMLE is probably one of the most difficult and complex exam you have to face in your professional life. So while most people have acquired enough study skills to pass and even do well in medical schools, the USMLE is altogether a different prospect and the better your study skills, the better you will fare in the exam.

In my experience, about 30% of people have enough study

and test-taking skills to do well in this exam. About another 30% have very poor study skills that they will either fail this exam or barely pass it by sheer luck. The other 40% although with adequate skills to pass and even do well on this exam, will actually fare better and get a higher score if they would just improve their study and test-taking skills. So, 7 out of 10 people taking the USMLE can actually improve their score by acquiring better studying skills.

What are the different Study Methods I need to learn for the USMLE

There are a variety of study methods, each of which will help you do your prep better. There are study methods that will help you understand what you are studying better. Other methods help you to retain information better. Others help your recall of information better. There are methods that improve your test taking ability and so on and so forth. We will tackle these various study skills and methods you can use to improve your performance individually.

Now, majority of the things you have to study in medicine are either a list of items or a process that you need to understand and memorize. In either case, there is a more efficient method of learning these things so that it is not only easier to memorize them, but you remember them in a way that makes it easier to answer questions in the exam. We will discuss this in detail later.

There are also certain things you need to know and skills you need to develop in order to make your studying more efficient. You need to know how to organize the topics you are studying so you not only can store information more efficiently, it can help you retrieve them much more easily when needed. Learning to read faster can help you study faster and in the exam go through questions faster. Practicing good retention and recall techniques throughout your review can improve the efficiency and effectiveness of your review.

How to Master the USMLE Step 1

Things you need to do throughout your review include mastering clinical vignettes and doing periodic assessment to assess your progress. You also need to integrate topics within a subject and between subjects throughout your review as a lot of questions in the USMLE involve integrated topics. ■

CHAPTER 13
LEARNING PHASE BASICS

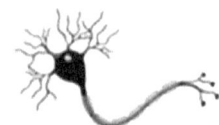

Purpose of the Learning Phase

The purpose of the Learning Phase is to study and understand all the medical concepts that will be tested in the USMLE. It is important to study and understand these concepts as it is very difficult to memorize and retain concepts you do not understand.

How we Learn

Pedagogy is the science of learning. However, based on the root word which comes from *pedia* as in pediatrics, it's actually the science of how children learn. Meanwhile, andragogy from the root word *andra* or man is the science of how adults learn. There is a big difference in the way adults learn vs. how children learn. Most people taking the USMLE are adults, whereas we started our medical education as young people barely out of childhood. Therefore a lot of learning skills we learned in school become less effective as we grow older. Hence, there is a need to learn how adults learn and adjust your study methods accordingly.

How to Master the USMLE Step 1

We will spend a few minutes discussing how we learn. Basically it starts during fetal development of the central nervous system. At birth, our CNS is composed of nerve cells with dendrites and axons that are not yet interconnected with each other. As we learn new things, these dendrites and axons form interconnections that remember what we have learned. These lack of interconnecting neurons at birth provide a limitless potential of what we can learn, however, it also means we know nothing at this stage and we lack skills. As we experience the world around us, these neurons form interconnections. The more we perform a certain task, or study a certain concept, the stronger the interconnections between the neurons responsible for that learning. These interconnections are usually formed while we sleep, that is why infants sleep longer than adults. Since they have a lot more to learn and need to form more interconnections than the typical adult.

However, starting at the age of 7 or thereabout, the human body starts eliminating unwanted neural interconnections and unused potential connections and strengthening connections that are already established. Strengthening of these interconnections increases the ability of the individual to carry out the actions mediated by these interconnections, at the expense of limiting the potential to learn new things. This is why language is usually learned best before age 7 and becomes increasingly difficult as we grow older. For example, there is no "L" sound in the Japanese language and older Japanese who learns English tends to pronounce L as R. But Japanese students who learn English at a young age have no problem pronouncing the L.

By age 21, these neural transformations are almost

over and it gets harder and harder to form new neural interconnections that are not in some way interconnected to neural pathways that are already formed. That is one of the main reasons that as we get older, it gets harder and harder to learn something really new. These changes have implications on how we learn.

As children, we usually learn by rote memorization. In fact if you remember how you were taught your ABC's and the multiplication tables, it's usually by sheer repetition. In fact a lot of times, we don't really understand what we were trying to memorize or why, just that we have to do them. As we grow older, we realize that understanding something can help us learn and memorize something faster. This is because learning something related to what you already know involves building neural interconnections to existing neural infrastructure rather than building something from scratch. As we grow older, we depend more and more on relationships to learn new things.

As children, we can memorize things without understanding, but as adults it is almost impossible to memorize anything without understanding them first. So you need to understand concepts before you memorize them and that is done using textbooks and lectures during the learning phase. You also need to relate any new concepts to what you already know so as to increase your recall of the concept. The more neural interconnections, the stronger the retention, the more interrelated the concepts you know to each other, the better the retention you have of all the concepts as a whole.

Materials to Use for the Learning Phase

The main study materials used in the learning phase

are textbooks and lectures, either audio, video or live. Textbooks provide detailed explanations, lots of examples and presume that you know very little of the topics discussed. Therefore, it is ideal to use textbooks if you do not understand the concepts to be tested yet. The main problem with textbooks is the length of the material itself, which makes it very hard to memorize and retain.

Lectures provide more focused explanations of the topics concerned and with live lectures, provide opportunities to ask questions and further explanations from resource persons. However, In order to memorize and retain details, you need repetition and the ability to focus specifically on materials you have not memorized. Therefore, lectures are not an ideal way to do that. You need to take down notes from the lectures and memorize that.

Recommended Study Materials for the Learning Phase

As we stated before, the best study materials for the learning phase are textbooks and lectures. Therefore we will discuss the various textbooks and recorded lectures that you can use during your learning phase.

For anatomy, NMS Clinical Anatomy or BRS Anatomy is enough for a basic understanding of Gross Anatomy. I still think that going for Gray's or Grant's Anatomy can be considered overkill, although if you really have forgotten anatomy, then you may need to use them. For Histology, BRS is more than adequate. Bloom and Fawcett is overkill although you may want to use it for the pics. For embryology, Langman's Embryology is more than enough, especially if you have forgotten most of embryology already.

For Physiology, Guyton or Ganong is more than adequate.

For Biochemistry, I recommend Lippincott's Illustrated Review of Biochemistry. Even though discussions there on Molecular Biology topics are practically non-existent, it is covered adequately in Pathology.

For Pathology, I still recommend that you use Robbin's Pathologic Basis of Diseases. Some people may complain that it is such a huge book and hard to study. But if you are serious about passing this exam or even doing well, believe me Big Robbins is indispensable. Make sure you pay special attention to Molecular Biology topics discussed in the cell pathology and neoplasia chapters as you need to tie them in with other molecular biology topics discussed in cell biology and physiology as well as in molecular genetics.

For Microbiology and Immunology, there is a good review book that can be used for the learning phase. Lange's Review of Microbiology and Immunology by Levinson i s very thorough in its discussion of concepts in microbiology and immunology. Therefore, going to a more basic textbook on microbiology and immunology is not really necessary.

For Pharmacology, Lippincott's Illustrated Review for Pharmacology is more than adequate for a review of the basics. It may not cover all the drugs, but it covers enough of the details of the prototype and principal drugs to make understanding it quite adequate.

How to Study the Learning Phase

The best way to approach the Learning Phase is to

study the subjects in the order it is taken in medical school. Remember in order to understand the medical concepts covered in Pathology, Microbiology and Immunology and Pharmacology, you need to know and understand topics covered in Anatomy, Physiology and Biochemistry.

Start by reading the recommended Anatomy and Physiology textbooks. What I would do is split my reading, anatomy in a.m. then physiology in p.m. That way it minimizes the boredom. It is important to study actively and that is best done by trying to explain aloud what you have just read to yourself, or write down notes, then reread the notes if it makes sense to you. Don't be afraid to use illustrations to help you understand the concepts. Drawing anatomical structures or creating diagrams of physiologic processes can help in understanding. Don't be afraid to reread topics you have read before so it can help you understand other concepts better.

Once you have finished reading both subjects, your next step is to integrate anatomy and physiology. Structure and function. For example, how does the anatomic structure of the lungs contribute to more efficient gas exchange? What specific cellular adaptations allow the lung to serve as a gas exchange mechanism? What about the kidneys? How does the structure of the nephron contribute to its function? Understanding structure and function correlation is important in understanding the basis of diseases and its treatment. If you do not do this right, then you will be forced to memorize the more advanced concepts in Pathology and even in clinical medicine without true understanding. That will severely handicap your ability to do well in the

USMLE as well as in medical practice.

You can start studying biochemistry at the same time as you start studying structure and function correlation. A significant portion of biochemistry can be studied alone but some topics are best correlated with corresponding topics in anatomy and physiology. For example, topics on metabolism and nutrition should be correlated with gastrointestinal physiology for better understanding. Genetics and Molecular Biology topics are best correlated with cell biology and cell physiology. Once you have finished the basics, you proceed to the more advanced topics like Pathology, Pharmacology and Microbiology/Immunology.

Integrate, Integrate, Integrate

The most important thing you need to do if you really want to do well in the USMLE is to integrate topics not only within a subject but also between subjects. Medicine is a very large discipline and it is very hard to understand everything all at once. It is best to break it into smaller pieces in order to digest them better. So we divide them into subjects and study them by subject. But after studying them piecemeal, like all the king's men, we need to put them back together again. We need to understand medicine as a whole in order to be able to make use of it in diagnosing and treating patients.

Most of you may have heard of the parable of the 7 blind men and the elephant. The first blind man who got hold of the elephant's trunk insists that the elephant is like a snake. The one who touched the ear insisted the elephant is like a large leaf. The one holding the legs insists the elephant is like a pillar while the one holding the elephant's torso was shouting loudly that an elephant is like a wall. Each was only partially right but on the whole wrong. And the only way they will truly understand what an elephant truly is, is to see it in its entirety.

So how do you do integration? First, you need to do integration within subject. For example, in anatomy: Whether you study them by system or by region, you need to understand how the different systems relate to one another. Then there are the sub-disciplines of anatomy like histology, embryology, etc. You now need to relate the gross structure to its microscopic features and its embryologic origins. For physiology, although you again study them by system, you need to understand that a lot of physiologic processes within a system affect other systems as well. And that some physiologic processes winds up affecting multiple systems instead.

In biochemistry, relating substrate metabolism with the chemical characteristics of the substrate being metabolized is an important step in the proper understanding of biochemistry. Understanding how these molecular substrates affects the different steps in their own metabolism is also crucial for doing well in this subject.

Integrating topics within pathology involves relating discussions in general pathology to systems pathology. General pathology discusses general pathologic processes applicable to most systems while systems pathology not only illustrates how these general pathologic processes manifest in individual systems, but also pathologic processes unique to each system. You need to understand how they relate to each other. There is also a need to integrate pathologic processes that occurs across systems.

Integrating within Microbiology and Immunology

also involves relating general characteristics of related organisms with specific characteristics of each organism. For example, discussions on Basic Bacteriology is related to general characteristics of Bacteria, including mode of transmission, life cycle, pathology, host reaction, treatment, etc. Clinical Bacteriology on the other hand deals with characteristics of specific Bacteria. Ditto for viruses, fungi and parasites.

Integrating within Pharmacology involves understanding how different subclasses of drugs are related to each other. Also, how the prototype drug of each subclass compare with other members of the same subclass.

After doing within subject integration, you need to do between subject integration. You need to integrate concepts within anatomy and physiology for structure and function correlation. Then integrate biochemical process into topics in both anatomy and physiology. The next step is to integrate all this into pathology.

Remember all pathologic processes are due to a disruption either in anatomic integrity, or physiologic or biochemical processes and the body's attempt either to compensate or restore this disruption. This compensation or restoration mechanism in turn has the potential to cause more disruptions. Then you need to integrate all these concepts to pharmacology.

Therapeutic interventions are designed to compensate or restore functions caused by pathology.

Pharmacotherapeutics is one modality you encounter in Step 1. Other modalities you encounter in Step 2 CK and Step 3. So you need to correlate Pharmacology back to physiology and biochemistry to understand how drugs work. And remember, these therapeutic interventions can, by themselves, cause their own pathology.

Microbiology and Immunology is a subject that is a good example of integration you need to do except it deal only with Infectious Disease. There are discussions in anatomy, physiology, biochemistry genetics, pathology and therapeutics all centered on infectious disease. Immunology is also discussed in this manner.

Advise to the Old IMG on the Learning Phase

The average person taking the USMLE Steps are fresh grads or third year medical students. Therefore understand that most of the prep course is geared towards these people and not to Old IMG. Therefore you need to be aware that you need to study differently from everyone else in order to pass this exam. More so if you want to do well.

The most important thing an old IMG need to do different from more recent grads is a formal Learning Phase. While recent grads still remember most of the basic science concepts, old IMG usually have forgotten a lot of the concepts and needs to relearn them. Recent grads can afford to skip a formal learning phase and proceed directly to the mastery phase. They can refer to textbooks when there is any material that they have forgotten and need to restudy. The reason they can do this is they still recall most of the concepts and needs to restudy only a few of them. For the old IMG who has forgotten most of these concepts, it's better to relearn everything first before memorizing them. ■

CHAPTER 14
WHAT TO DO DURING MASTERY PHASE

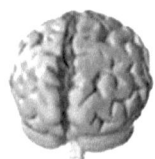

Purpose of the Mastery Phase

The purpose of the Mastery Phase is to be able to memorize, retain and recall concepts tested by the USMLE at the right level of detail required by the exam. One mistake a lot of people make in studying for the USMLE is thinking that just understanding the topics tested is enough to do well in the USMLE. Nothing is farther from the truth. The USMLE requires you not only to understand the topics tested but to be able to recall the details very fast.

The Devil is in the Details

Far too many times, the number one complaint people have when answering online q banks is this: "I know the concept being tested by the question. I know I have read this topic numerous times. But I can't seem to find the answer." The reason the person is having this problem is that he did not memorize the concepts at the right level of detail required for the exam. Not all concepts are treated equally by the USMLE. Some concepts you just need to understand the basics and you can answer the questions. For others you need to know every detail about the topic in order to be able to answer the question. Not being able to recall the topic in the right level of detail can cause you to fail to answer the question.

Part of the Mastery Phase is that you make sure you memorize the topics in the right amount of detail for the exam. You need to make sure the study materials you are using cover everything in the right amount of detail. Failure to do so can affect your final results. The course is set up to ensure that you cover the right level of detail for the exam.

The Need for Speed

One of the things most student taking the USMLE underestimate about this exam is how little time they have to answer each questions. On average you have about 1 minute and 20 seconds for each question. You have to read the question, understand it, recall what you know about the topic being asked, do any analysis needed, go through the choices, work through any distractors or two to three step thinking built into the answer choices, then choose the answer. Therefore, you need to give yourself every advantage you need during the exam itself. And the best time to insure that you have the necessary skill and covered whatever weak point you have is during prep time.

So what do you need to do to speed up your overall test taking ability?

5.   **Learn to Read Fast.** The faster you finish reading the question, the more time you have to think about the answer. Remember by the last 3 blocks, your brain is tired and you will be reading slower than when you started the exam. If you are reading slowly from the start, you will be glacial by the time you reach the last few blocks. We will discuss how to train yourself to read faster in later sections.

6. **Practice moving from question to question fast.** A bad habit people have is moving slowly to the next question. They do that during practice and expect they can speed up during the actual exam. Nothing is farther from the truth. How fast you go thru questions is a matter of habit. You can temporarily will yourself to answer questions faster. But if you are concentrating on speeding up, it distracts you from thinking about the answer. Once you start concentrating on thinking about the answer, habit takes over and you automatically slow down. You need to practice speed and the course includes speed-building practice in answering questions.

7. **Anticipate questions during your prep.** For every question that you have anticipated that will come out in the exam, that is one less question you need to spend an inordinate amount of time thinking through during the exam. You know the answer right away and can move fast to the next one. But how do you know what questions will come out in the exam. Most people actually go through various q banks and even the NBME assessment tests, hoping somehow they can find some questions there that will come out in the exam. Some asked their friends or classmates who have taken the exam for tips. There are various ways to anticipate what questions will come out in the exam and they will be discussed throughout the course.

8. **Do analysis during prep to minimize the need for analysis during the exam.** Analyzing and correlating concepts take time. And in a timed exam like the USMLE, time is a commodity you are always short of. Therefore, try to make your analysis and correlation during the prep process. Compared to the time you have during the exam, you have all the time in the world during prep time. Part of the effectiveness of Goljan's pathology lectures in raising scores is that it

does the correlation and analysis of some of the more important topics during the lecture. So answering questions on the exam itself is just a matter of remembering the results of those analysis and correlation rather than doing the analysis and correlation during the exam.

9. **Make sure you can recall what you have memorized very fast.** The best way to memorize and retain information is to study them in an organized manner. Organization of the concepts can make it easier for you to relate them to each other increasing retention. However, the nature of the USMLE requires you to recall the information in a random manner and you need to be able to recall them fast. We will discuss ways to improve retention and recall in other sections of this book.

Study Materials to Use for the Mastery Phase

The best types of materials to use for the Mastery Phase are notes and reviewers, rather than textbooks or lectures. Mastery is about memorizing and being able to recall those information. Textbooks are too long to memorize and not necessary. Lectures, unless in note form, are also impossible to memorize. Notes and reviewers are in the form of bulleted lists, tables, illustrations, etc. They are the same information you find in textbooks and lectures but in more compact form.

Technically, notes can be divided into two forms although very few notes conform to these two forms. I call them study notes and outline notes.

Study notes are notes that are written in a more detailed format. It covers both high yield and low yield topics that may come out in the examination. It is still written in the form of bulleted lists, tables and illustrations, but with occasional explanatory notes to clarify more difficult concept which the author may want the reader to understand. It differs from textbooks in that there is little by way of explaining the concepts or giving examples. Examples of study notes include the Kaplan Lecture Notes and NMS series of Reviewers.

Outline notes on the other hand are very compact version of study notes, focusing mostly on high yield materials. It presumes you know the materials being tested already and is just doing a very quick review in order to insure last minute retention of the most important facts before sitting for the exam. You should not use outline notes alone if there are a lot of topics that you do not know or have not done a formal prep. Examples of outline notes are First Aid for the USMLE Step 1, High Yield Series and Board Review Series. Board Review Series is actually kind of hybrid. It is more than just an outline note but fall short of being a study note.

On the course, there are both study notes and outline notes for your use. Use the study notes throughout your prep, switching to the outline notes when you switch to high yield review.

For improving recall, flashcards are probably one of the best tools you can use. However, don't use the commercially available flashcards. They are designed for studying the topics concerned and not for improving random recall. It's best to make your own flashcards or use the available online flashcards on my prep site. The best flashcards to improve recall should only contain one point or topic per card. For example, a card should only contain Staphylococcus Aureus, treatment of choice and not a full description of S. Aureus. S. Aureus Disease belongs to another card, etc.

Recommended Study Materials for the Mastery Phase

The following are the recommended study materials for the mastery phase. Please read through the discussions of how to review the individual subject in order to understand how to use the study materials properly If you plan to use other study materials, make sure you pass them by me first to make sure it is appropriate for use.

Pathology study notes:

- *Askdoc's Pathology Study Notes*
- Kaplan Pathology Lecture Notes

Pathology outline notes:

- *Askdoc's Pathology Outline Notes*
- BRS Pathology

Pathology supplement:

- *Goljan's Rapid Review of Pathology*
- Goljan's audio lecture and notes

Pathology per chapter quiz book:

- *Robbin's Review of Pathology*

Pharmacology study notes:

- *Askdoc's Pharmacology Study Notes**
- *Illustrated Review of Pharmacology*
- *Katzung's Review of Pharmacology*
- Kaplan Pharmacology Lecture Notes

Pharmacology outline notes:

- *Askdoc's Pharmacology Outline Notes**

Pharmacology per chapter quiz:

- *Katzung's Review of Pharmacology*

Microbiology and Immunology study notes:

- *Askdoc's Microbiology and Immunology Study Notes*
- *Review of Microbiology and Immunology by Jawetz*
- Kaplan Microbiology and Immunology Lecture

Notes

Microbiology and Immunology outline notes:

- *Askdoc's Microbiology and Immunology Outline Notes**

Microbiology and Immunology per chapter quiz:

- *Review of Microbiology and Immunology by Jawetz*

For the minor 4 subjects (Anatomy, Physiology, Biochemistry and Behavioral Sciences) there are no per chapter quizzes. You can use Kaplan's Q Book for this purpose. Behavioral Sciences use only one type of notes.

Gross Anatomy study notes:

- *Askdoc's Gross Anatomy Study Notes**
- *Kaplan's Anatomy Lecture Notes*
- BRS Gross Anatomy
- NMS Gross Anatomy

Gross Anatomy outline notes:

- *Askdoc's Gross Anatomy Outline Notes**
- *High Yield Gross Anatomy*

Neuroanatomy study notes:

- *Askdoc's Neuroanatomy Study Notes**
- Kaplan's Anatomy Lecture Notes
- *BRS Neuroanatomy*

Neuroanatomy outline notes:

- *Askdoc's Neuroanatomy Outline Notes**
- *High Yield Neuroanatomy*

Histology/Embryology study notes:

- *Askdoc's Histology/Embryology Study*

How to Master the USMLE Step 1

Notes*
- *Kaplan's Anatomy Lecture Note*
- Lange's Embryology
- BRS Cell Biology

Histology/Embryology outline notes:

- *Askdoc's Histology/Embryology Outline Notes**

Physiology study notes:

- *Askdoc's Physiology Study Notes**
- *Kaplan's Physiology Lecture Notes*

Physiology outline notes:

- *Askdoc's Physiology Outline Notes**
- *BRS Physiology*

Biochemistry study notes:

- *Askdoc's Biochemistry Study Notes**
- *Illustrated Review of Biochemistr*
- *Kaplan's Biochemistry Lecture Notes*

Biochemistry outline notes:

- *Askdoc's Biochemistry Outline Notes**

Behavioral Sciences notes:

- *Askdoc's Behavioral Sciences Notes**
- *BRS Behavioral Sciences*
- Kaplan's Behavioral Sciences Lecture Notes.

For flashcards, it is not recommended to buy commercially available flashcards. Either use the available online flashcards on my prep site or make your own. For advice on how to make your own flashcards for each subject, refer to the sections on how to review for each of the subjects.

How to Study for the Mastery Phase

I'll be giving a general overview on how to study for the Mastery Phase. Please refer to individual sections for more detailed discussions of the topics mentioned in this section.

The main purpose of the Mastery Phase is to memorize, retain and be able to recall the topics being tested by the exam at the right level of detail for the exam. In order to do this, first you need to make sure that you are using study materials that cover all the topics that will come out in the exam at the right level of detail. Next you need to be able to memorize these materials and recall them fast enough for the purpose of the exam.

First, the material you are studying should cover not only the topics on each subject, but all the integration, correlations and analysis that will come out in the exam. Just knowing the facts of each topic and given enough time, you will be able to use these topics to correlate, integrate and analyze the questions during the exam. But given the fact that this is the USMLE, and time is the commodity we are always in short supply on, you need to make sure you cover all the integration, correlation and analysis you need during prep time in order to insure that you need to do as little of this time-consuming stuff during the examination itself.

Second, in order to insure that you can maximize your ability to retain and recall information as well as do them rapidly, the way you memorize and retain this information is a very important factor. Fast recall also needs to be practiced often so it becomes second nature to you.

The course is designed to help you achieve this. Therefore it is important to follow the methodology of the course, not just the topics being covered. The methodologies of the course are designed to maximize your study efficiency, improve your ability to retain and recall information and help you answer questions better. But you need to follow the methods. Just enrolling in the course and then merrily reviewing using your own methods will not do that. And yet you will be surprised at how many people do just that and wonder why they don't do that well.

The first thing we need to establish is that you will need a minimum of three revisions in order to insure you have a reasonable chance of passing this exam much less do well. And by three revisions, I don't mean reading three times. Each revision has a goal. For some people, they can read the material once and reach that goal. For others it takes more than reading once, some even five times to finish one revision. Therefore, you need to assess your ability in order to know how many times you need to read through the material in order to achieve 3 revisions. Read up on the section on doing three revisions for details on how to do this.

The next thing we need to do is to learn how to memorize the various things you need to memorize. Majority of things you need to memorize in Step 1 can be divided into two. A list of items you need to memorize or processes you need to study and memorize. There are specific ways to study and memorize lists that will not only make it easier to retain and recall them; it will also help you anticipate the possible questions that will come out in the exam. The same holds true for studying processes. Studying processes the right way not only helps you retain and recall them better, you can anticipate questions that will come out in the exam and help you integrate topics between subject better. For more detailed explanations on how to do this, read up on the sections about memorizing list of items and studying processes.

Right from the start, you need to ensure that you are doing periodic assessment to monitor your progress. The most common mistakes people do is to go straight into review and the first time they assess their progress is when they do the q bank and find out that they made little progress in the past two to three months of their prep. By doing periodic assessment right from the start, you ensure you are studying the correct way and progressing steadily.

The second most common mistake people do is to use either the NBME self assessment tests or the online q bank themselves to monitor their progress. The best use of the NBME self assessment tests is to gauge your readiness to sit for the actual exam itself. Using them to monitor your progress actually wastes the tests because you are presuming once you have gone through all the forms; you are ready for the exam. What if you still aren't and you are forced to study further, what then would you use to monitor your progress? Don't make that mistake.

Online q banks on the other hand are best used to learn how to answer USMLE type questions. At the start of your prep, you are concentrating on learning and memorizing concepts. Therefore, answering questions at that time helps you with remembering concepts, not training you to answer tough questions. Only when you know the concepts can you concentrate on learning how to answer tough USMLE type questions. If you use online q banks right at the start of your prep, by the time you are trying to learn how to answer tough questions, you run out of q banks. Read up on the section on Periodic Assessment to find out how to do this right.

One of the best ways to ensure that you study everything and be able to retain and recall information better and faster is to study the topics in an organized manner. By organizing information together into headings and subheadings, you can be sure if you covered everything you need to study or not. Also as you go through the long prep process, you encounter new information that is somehow related to information you already know. You can link them together under the same heading in your head, making it easier to retain and recall. And lastly, each question in the USMLE usually pertains to a specific topic under a specific heading or subheading. If you can isolate the specific topic covered by the question, then you know the correct answer is limited to topics under that specific heading or subheading. Read up on how to organize topics in the appropriate section.

With the clinical slant of the USMLE even for Step 1, there is a need to pay attention to clinical vignettes. A large portion of the questions you will encounter in the exam is in the form of clinical vignettes. In order to be able to answer the question, you need to be able to diagnose the case. If you are unable to diagnose it, you won't be able to answer the question, even if you know the answer if the diagnosis was given to you. Read up on Mastering Clinical Vignettes for more detail on how to do this.

Lastly, it is very important to do a high yield review a week or two before sitting for the exam. Notice I am not advocating a high yield review only prep as a lot of people have mistakenly done. Doing just a high yield review for this exam can lead to disastrous results. However, it is important to do a high yield review after you have done a full prep but just before you sit for the exam. It could add a lot of points to your final score. Read up on High Yield Review to find out how to do this.

Integration for the Mastery Phase

Integrating for the Mastery Phase is slightly different from integrating for the Learning Phase. Whereas, during the Learning Phase, you concentrate on learning and understanding how the various subjects integrate within each other and between each other, during the Mastery Phase, the concentration is on being able to retain and recall those integrated topics at the right level of detail for the exam.

CHAPTER 15
DOING 3 REVISIONS FOR MASTERY

Why Do 3 Revisions

Very few people can pass this exam, more so do well with less than 3 revisions. In my assessment, it is next to impossible to pass this exam with just one revision. A few can pass it with 2 revisions, but most will need 3 or more revisions. You may have heard that some people were able to pass the exam with just 1 revision. Actually most of them would probably be third year medical students. Most American medical schools would have prepped their students for the exam before they start reviewing on their own. And for most of them, they just covered the subjects being tested a few months before. So what they claim is just one revision is actually multiple revisions. Of course, there are people who actually lie, especially in forums.

In general the more revisions you do the higher the score you will achieve. The reason is that repetition is the surest way to remember anything you study. But learning by repetition is time consuming and therefore, relying on repetition alone is usually not recommended. Plus, everyone eventually burns out if the prep period is prolonged. So it's important to make sure that each revision you do is effective and achieve the goal you have set, so you can get the maximum score you are able in as few revisions as possible.

Purpose of Each Revision

Every revision has its purpose and goal you need to achieve. Insuring you fulfil the purpose and achieve the goal set is important in order to minimize mistakes and avoid unnecessarily prolonging your prep.

The purpose of the first revision is to memorize and recall the topics of each subject. There are general methods of doing this and will be discussed subsequently. It is important to do integration within the same subject during this time. Each subject is too large to discuss in one go, so they are usually divided into chapters. You need to correlate and integrate these chapters so you understand the subject as a whole.

For example, Pathology is generally divided into General Pathology and Systems Pathology. General Pathology discusses general principles of pathologic processes that apply to all tissues in general and make comparisons when there are variations to these processes. When we reach Systems Pathology, discussions revolve around pathologic processes that are specific to each system and tissues belonging to those systems. You now need to relate the general processes to the specific processes in each system and be aware of the differences. Why? Because the USMLE will test whether you know the difference between these processes or not.

You also need to ensure that you are retaining the information you are studying and will be able to recall what you have read and memorized. Therefore it is important that you take assessment of your progress and make sure you have retained enough information before moving on to the next subject.

How to Master the USMLE Step 1

For the second revision, the main purpose is to integrate the different subjects together. Medicine is a very large discipline, so it is very hard to learn everything all at once. It is divided into subjects so it becomes easier to learn and absorb. However, the effect of that is your knowledge of medicine becomes fragmented. Like all the king's horses and all the king's men you need to put humpty dumpty back together again. A large portion of the USMLE tests whether you have integrated the different topics together and understand them as such. Thus failure to integrate all the subjects can result in doing poorly in this exam.

You still continue to memorize the topics under each subject, but you also need to memorize and be able to recall the topics you have integrated. What you can do is write anything you have integrated in the margin of your notes. This is to insure that, when you do your third revision, you pay attention to these integrated topics too.

For the third revision, the main purpose is to cover whatever weak points you still have. Even if you studied everything in the first two revisions, you will always have weak points. The reason is that not all topics interest us. Topics we find interesting, we pay special attention to. Topics we find boring, we tend to tune out. So even if you are reading those topics, your eyes may be seeing the words but your mind will tend to wander. However, the USMLE tests for topics that are important for clinical practice and not whether it interests you or not. So you need to cover those weak points.

You do your third revision at the same time as you start online q banks. The reason is that you use the online q banks to find your weak points and cover them. You continue to review everything however, including integrated topics. But whatever weak points you have as pointed out by your results on the q bank, you need to do additional revisions.

After doing the three revisions, there is still one thing you need to do to insure you will do well. Some call it a fourth revision, but actually it's not a full revision. I call it a high yield review. At this stage you are only about two to three weeks from sitting for the exam. You concentrate on insuring you remember all the high yield materials that have a big chance of coming out in the exam. The mistake of a lot of people is thinking that they only need a high yield review to pass this exam. The mistake a lot of people think about my course is that you don't do a high yield review at all. Now you know that you have to. If your school has done a proper prep for you already, you can skip all the three revisions and go directly to high yield review.

How to Do the 3 Revisions

We will discuss in general how to do each of the revisions properly. More detailed discussions of specific methods are discussed under various topics on how to study. Detailed discussion of what to do on each subject on each revision are discussed under the sections on how to review each of the subject.

For the first revision, we need to memorize, retain and be able to recall the topics within a subject. We also need to be able to integrate the different topics within a subject.

The first step we need to be able to do is understand how the subject is organized and memorize the headings and subheadings. This will give you the necessary framework to relate the different topics within a subject together and remember them better. Read in more detail on how and why you need to organize topics in the section on organizing topics.

Next, there are basically two types of information that covers most of what you need to study in your prep. Either you have a list of items that you need to memorize or you have a process that you need to understand and memorize. There is a very effective way to study for both and yet it's surprising that most people do not study them that way. You can read up on how to study lists and processes under the specific headings.

But in general, you study lists by first memorizing the items of a list. Only then do you study the details of each item and compare them with each other. Take note of what is different and what is the same because that is what will come out in the exam most often. When you study processes, you study all the steps of the processes first and understand how each step relates to each other. Only then do you study the details of each step and take note of how any changes, disruption or modification of this step will affect the process as whole and other steps in the same process and other processes.

Also take note that most of what you will have to study will be variations of the above. Details of items in a list can be composed of another list or processes. Details of steps in the process can be another process or a list of items. This can go on for several iterations, so study them as is.

While doing your prep, you will notice that you may encounter the same topic multiple times and in different context. It will be a big mistake to think that it's a waste of time to go through them again and that you can skip the topic that you have encountered before. The reason you need to study them again is that questions can come from different contexts and studying them in one context does not necessarily mean you can answer questions about the same topic if presented in a different context.

A good example is anti-bacterial drugs. You can study them from the context of Microbiology, i.e. organisms and what drugs affect them. Or you can study them from the context of Pharmacology, i.e. drugs and organisms they affect. The USMLE can ask the question from either context. If you study them only from one context, say Microbiology and the question is presented in the other context say Pharmacology, you may have difficulty getting the answer immediately and in some cases fail to get the answer at all. For example, you studied *Streptococcus Pneumoniae* and you know that drug of choice is ampicillin or amoxicillin. Alternate drugs include erythromycin, clarithromycin, azithromycin, etc. if the question starts with the organism and what drugs are effective; you won't have problems answering the question. On the other hand, if the drug is given, say azithromycin and you are asked which organisms are susceptible, you will be forced to recall by organism then what drugs affect them. And if you miss one, you miss the question. If during review, you took the time to memorize the organisms susceptible to each drug, i.e. in both contexts, either way the question comes out, you got it.

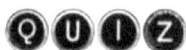

Another important thing you should be doing is per chapter quiz at least for the big three. This will insure that you are retaining enough materials as you finish each chapter before moving on to the next one. That way you can correct any problem with your study methods right from the start. In the course, we put a minimum passing score of 80% for each chapter. Doing per chapter quiz for the minor four is optional. But you should do a per subject quiz after you finish each subject.

Lastly, during your first revision, you will notice that there will still be topics that you do not fully understand. When this happens, it is very important that you go back to textbooks to understand those topics. For a list of textbooks you can use for this purpose, please go to the section on Learning Phase basics.

For the second revision, you need to start integrating the subjects together. You will still continue to memorize each of the subjects as you did in your first revision, although you will be able to do this much more quickly this time. Do your integration. You can write them as notes on the margin of your study notes. For more detailed discussions on how to integrate between subjects, go to the appropriate section.

At this point you should also start improving your ability to recall what you have studied. This is best done using flashcards. Online flashcards are available on the course. Or you can make your own. Go to specific discussions on each of the subject to find out how to build your own flashcards. Don't buy those commercial flashcards currently available in the market. I bought them but never really got to use them.

For the course, there is a q bank software we use for speed building exercise. You also start them at this point of your prep. If you are not in the course, I recommend you get the rapid review series of question bank for this purpose. In the speed building exercise, you try to go through each question as fast as possible. Try to finish 4 questions per minute. At this stage, it is more important to finish fast than to get a high score. Eventually your score will go up.

For the third revision, the concentration will be

identifying your weak areas and do extra reviews on them. You will still continue to memorize the subjects, this time also covering the integrated topics you have put on your marginal notes. However, you have started doing online q banks at this point. So you should have an idea where your weak points are using the results of the online q banks as guide. For details on how to use the q banks, read the section on using online q banks under Test Preparation Strategy. When you have identified a specific weak point, it is important to cover the topics again even if you have finished covering it in your prep.

Lastly, just two weeks before you sit for the exam, you need to do at least one high yield review. For the high yield review, you have the choice of using my online high yield notes, First Aid for the USMLE or my online High Yield Fast Facts. The purpose of this high yield review is to make sure that what you remember the most are the really high yield stuff. ■

CHAPTER 16
HIGH YIELD REVIEW

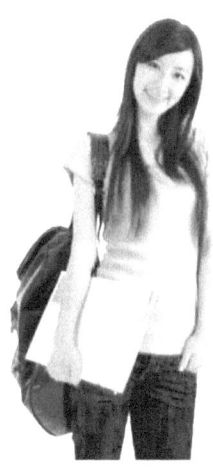

Why Do a High Yield Review

It is important to understand that about 2/3 of the exam will be about high yield materials. Therefore it is important that you master the high yield materials in order that you have a good chance of passing this exam or even doing well and scoring high. It is also important to understand that high yield materials comprise at most 20 to 25% of all materials that can come out in the exam proper. Therefore by making sure you have mastered the high yield materials, you can get a higher score while studying less.

That said, there is a caveat. If you study high yield materials only, no matter how well you mastered them, there is a good chance that you will fail this exam and it is almost impossible to do well. You still need to cover the lower yield stuff. In fact the best way to score high is to master all the high yield stuff and memorize as much lower yield stuff as you are able without forgetting the high yield stuff.

One of the favourite study plans very popular in a lot of forums is to do a high yield review then follow it up with an online q bank. Make notes of the questions you were unable to answer in the q bank and review them just before the exam. This plan can and does work, but it can cause you to score lower than what you might achieve if you did the prep right. The reason this can happen is because studying this way violates the principle of recency as one of the three R's of retention and recall. The more recently you encounter particular information, the stronger you are able to recall that information. Since you did a high yield review first, the questions you encountered in the online q banks that you did not understand are mostly lower yield topics. By reviewing them instead of the high yield topics so very near the exam date, you run the risk of forgetting high yield stuff in favour of lower yield materials. You can offset this problem by doing a high yield review just before sitting for the exam.

In the course, you avoid these problem altogether. You start by studying everything that might come out in the exam both high yield and low yield stuff. As your prep progress, you start concentrating on higher yield stuff. When you hit the online q banks, you will tend to score higher as you know a lot of the lower yield stuff you encounter in the q banks. Then you do a final high yield review just before sitting for the exam.

Recognizing High Yield Topics

The question of course is how do you recognize high yield topics? There is no foolproof way to know all the high yield topics and how high yield a topic is, is relative. But there are certain parameters you can use to guide you on choosing the high yield stuff. You can of course depend on the reviewers that discuss only high yield topics to find out what is high yield. But eventually you will discover that although for the most part, people agree on what is high yield; there are significant differences between review book authors. Plus if you are aiming for a high score, you probably need to make an assessment on what you need to study more yourself.

First, we need to understand that the mandate of the USMLE is to test our readiness to practice clinical medicine in the United States. Majority of medical students will wind up in clinical practice with only a small minority in academic and research medicine. Therefore expect a clinical slant in the exam even if Step 1 is all about basic sciences. Therefore, any topic that has clinical applications will be higher yield. For example, knowing how to use and interpret diagnostic tests is more high-yield than how to do it step by step. Another example are cancer chemotherapeutic drugs. You will need to know the drugs and on what cancers they are basically effective but you don't need to know the different combination of specific drugs for specific cancers as they change continually and best left to specialists.

Second, we need to understand that the USMLE wants to know if you understand Medicine, not just if you have memorized it. In Step 1, this means understanding mechanisms of disease i.e. pathophysiology. Understanding different biological processes and how disease occurs through disruption of these processes. Knowing the difference between two concepts and differentiating different diseases from each other. Therefore, it is important to know the difference between similar concepts. A simple example is the different types of necrosis. Can you easily distinguish between coagulation necrosis, liquefactive necrosis, caseous necrosis, etc? In pharmacology an example is being able to differentiate between various subclasses of drugs that basically do the same thing. Take diuretics, they all cause diuresis, but the different subclasses are different in the way they accomplish this and their diuretic effects. The USMLE will test if you know the difference.

Lastly, it is important to understand that topics can't really be neatly divided into high yield and low yield. It's actually a spectrum. There are very high yield topics and very low yield topics and a lot in between. You know you have to cover very high yield topics and you can ignore very low yield topics. But those in between is a judgment call. That is part of the reason you use reviewers, since they represent what other people think are high yield, especially the high yield reviewers like First Aid, High Yield Series and BRS series of reviewers. Or enrol in a prep course like this one.

How to do a High Yield Review

The best way to start your high yield review is two to three weeks before you sit for the exam and after you have finished your main prep. The best material to use is the outline notes provided in the course. Good alternatives are high yield reviewers like First Aid, High Yield Series or some of the BRS reviewers.

When doing your high yield review, don't just read through them like some people are wont to do. Try to memorize them, recite them out loud so you can recall them. Take note of illustrations and how to identify them. Draw out any process whether physiologic, biochemical or pathologic to remember them better. It is highly recommended that you do flashcards to improve your recall. In the course we use the online flashcards in my site like High Yield Fast Facts for this purpose. ∎

CHAPTER 17
HOW TO MEMORIZE LIST OF ITEMS

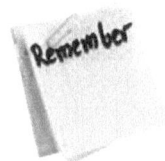

How People Normally Memorize a List of Items

Normally given a list of item to memorize, people will memorize it in the order that is presented. To illustrate, suppose you are to memorize a list of items from 1 to 6 with subitems a to e. Most people will start by memorizing item 1a, 1b, 1c and so on and so forth. Then they proceed to memorize item 2a, 2b, 2c, etc. You will see later why this is not the right way to memorize a list of items.

Askdoc's Method of Memorizing a List of Items

Now the method I recommend you use to memorize the same list of items is this. First memorize items 1 to 6 noting that they belong to the same group of information. Then once you are able to recite item 1 to 6 in order, proceed to memorize all the items in item 1, i.e. item 1a, item 1b, etc.

Once you have finished memorizing item 1 proceed to memorizing item 2 details. However, it is important for you to do this one extra step; compare the details between item 1 and item 2 and ask yourself, how they are the same and how they are different. Take note of the differences and memorize what is different between item 1 and item 2. Then do this again with item 3 comparing it first to item 1 then to item 2.

Why Use My Method to Memorize a List of Items

Now, you may wonder why my method is superior to the other method. It is important to understand that the USMLE rarely asks a question that all you need you do is just recall what is memorized. It presumes you have already memorized all that information. What it wants to know is do you know the difference between two concepts and majority of the questions in the USMLE is of that type.

So imagine if you get a question that requires you to differentiate between Item 1 and 2 of the example above. It could be as simple as diagnosing if you are dealing with a case of squamous cell carcinoma of the lung or bronchioalveolar carcinoma. If you memorized it using the first method, you will first need to remember all the features of item 1, i.e. item 1a, item 1b, etc. Then you need to recall all the details of item 2. Then you need to compare the details between item 1 and item 2 and look for what's different so you can make the diagnosis. If you have to do that during the exam, then you have around a minute to do all of that. Now, if you forgot even 1 detail of item 1 or item 2 and that happens to be the difference, you are in big trouble. Another problem is when it turns out you need to do three different comparisons to answer one question and you realize how much problem you will have using the first method.

Now differentiating between item 1 and 2 using the second method is actually better. When you encounter the same question and you need to differentiate between item 1 and 2, you first go through the list in your head on the difference between the 2 items, which you did when you were memorizing. It's faster and surer then having to go thru two lists and find the answer there. Now if you forgot what the difference is, only then do you need to go through item 1 and its details and then item 2 and its details and compare to note the difference. So actually you have two chances of getting the correct answer instead of just one. Plus if you need to do three or more comparisons to answer just one question you will realize that you can save a lot of time doing it this way.

Some people will complain that it takes more time and effort to study this way. But as we discussed earlier, any time you save in the actual exam is crucial. Increasing your study time 25 to 30% in exchange for cutting your time answering questions by 20 to 50% is well worth the effort. Compared to the time you have in the exam, your time for prepping is actually almost limitless. What you are doing here is analyzing and making comparisons during review so you don't have to do it during the exam when your time is very limited. As we said before, for the USMLE, only what happens on exam day really counts, so anything you can do to make sure your performance is at its peak during exam day, the better. ■

CHAPTER 18
HOW TO STUDY PROCESSES

How People Normally Study Processes

Processes are the second most common type of concept we need to study. Processes are commonly used to describe how things work. Most concepts in physiology and biochemistry involve processes. Pathophysiology concepts are mostly processes, too. Processes are usually composed of steps and description of each step of the process. Under each step could be a list of items to memorize or another description of a process.

Most people normally study processes, this way. First, they memorize the first step. Then they study the details of the first step. They then proceed to memorize the second step, then the details of the second step and so on and so forth. Until they finish the whole process. There are however, a lot of disadvantages in studying processes this way.

First, you never see the whole picture. You study each step in isolation of other steps and never see the process as a whole. A lot of questions in the USMLE will focus on your understanding of the process as whole rather than individual steps.

Second, it is not clear-cut how each step is related to the next step. Studying each step in isolation also prevents you from seeing how each step affect another step in the process. A step can affect other steps immediately before or after it or steps a few steps away.

Third, there are a limited number of ways a step affect another step and even though there may be 30 step in a process, there will be at most 4 to 5 ways they affect each other. If you study steps in isolation, you will have to memorize all 30 steps individually rather than studying them in related groups. This takes more time.

Askdoc's Method of Studying Processes

Given the above problems, how should you study processes? The best way to study processes is this way. First, memorize all the steps of the process in the proper order. Next, study the details of each step. Then you need to understand how each step affects the step before and after it.

Also understand that products of any step in the process can affect other steps in the process in varying ways.

- They could enhance or retard the step providing positive feedback.

- They could enhance or retard the step providing negative feedback.

- They could modify the step, changing the product of that step.

The way to deal with this is after studying the whole process, as discussed earlier: take the extra step of grouping the steps according to the effects of the steps on other steps. Group steps with positive feedback together and study them together. Then group together steps with negative feedback and so on and so forth. You will find examples of how to do these on the discussions on how to review individual subjects.

Why Use My Method to Study Processes

The USMLE is a timed exam. In fact, the one thing you are always short of in the USMLE is time. Therefore, anything you do that will save time in the USMLE exam itself will help improve the outcome tremendously.

First, most questions in the USMLE will test whether you understand the process as a whole.

Second, they will also test if you know how each step of the process affects the other step.

Lastly, all diseases, drugs, hormones and enzymes act on those steps and therefore understanding those steps will help you learn them better.

Studying processes in order to make sure you cover the above considerations require tremendous amount of analysis to be done during your revision. However, if you do not do this during your review, you need to do this during the exam itself. And as we said before, time is the commodity in shortest supply during the exam. Compared to the exam proper itself where you have just over a minute to read the question, recall the topic concerned, make your analysis and answer the question, the time you have during your prep is virtually unlimited.

By doing your analysis during your review, you minimize the amount of analysis you do during the exam. Recalling the result of your analysis during prep is several orders faster than trying to do the analysis during the exam.■

CHAPTER 19

ORGANIZING TOPICS: ORGANIZING HEADINGS AND SUBHEADINGS

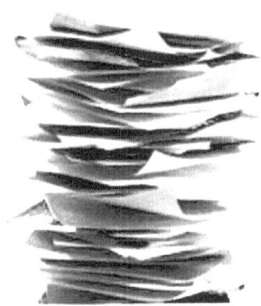

Why You Need to Organize Topics

One of the best ways you can improve your ability to retain and recall information is to organize them into topics. It will help you to remember things better and more efficiently. It will help you to integrate new information to what you already know. It will also help you narrow down and find the correct answer during the exam itself.

How to Organize Topics in Your Prep

Throughout the course, we make use of the chapters in our notes to organize what we learn. In order to make use of these chapter headings and subheadings, we need to take the time to memorize them so we can use them as outline to organize what we know and what we will learn throughout the review.

It also makes sense to organize your topics for Anatomy, Physiology and Biochemistry around the relevant topics of Pathology. This way, it makes it easier to recall even the integrated topics you have studied and memorized.

If you are using reference materials outside of my notes, you need to organize them yourself. Usually following the chapters for your main heading will suffice. But the subheadings may require some thinking through. Group similar information together. If two items can be compared and contrasted, pair them under the same subheadings, easier to remember that way. If you are aiming for a high score, there may be some lower yield information you want to memorize to give you an advantage. Group them together so easier to find them in subsequent review.

What to Do When You Encounter New Information about a Topic

One of the main reasons it makes sense to organize what you have studied into topics is that it is easier to incorporate new information about those topic to information you already know. A lot of times when you are studying, you encounter related information at various times of your prep and not all at the same time. When situation like that arises, you need to be able to incorporate that knowledge into what you already know and not just memorize it as a singular piece of information unrelated to the rest.

Usually you will encounter new information if you use more than one text or reviewer for each subject in your prep. Coverage of each reference material is usually different in some respect and you may encounter new material about the same topic. Another time when you can encounter new information is while doing the online q banks. Therefore you need a method to incorporate this information effectively.

The way to file it appropriately organized in your head is to do it this way. When you encounter new information, try to integrate with what you already know about that topic. Does this information match what I already know? Does it contradict what I know? Does it clarify what I know? Does it modify what I know?

Once you have done the integration it will be much, much easier to remember the new information later.

Narrowing Down and Finding the Answers to Questions

During the exam proper, you need to have mastered the USMLE enough that you can find the answer immediately after reading the question. You need to be able to do this for at least 1/3 to 1/2 the questions in the exam or you run the risk of running out of time to finish the exam.

However, no matter how much you try to memorize everything, you will not be able to do that for every question. There will be times when after reading the question, the answer remains elusive. When that happens, you need a systematic way of finding the answer. Just groping in the dark wastes valuable time. That's when the time you invested in organizing and memorizing those organized topics will pay off.

We need to understand that every question in the USMLE revolves around one topic. Therefore, when you encounter a question and the answer does not come to you immediately, the first step you need to do is see what topic the question is all about. Then try to remember all the information you know about that topic. You will realize then that the correct answer will revolve around the topic. When you go through the choices, eliminate any choice that is not covered by the topic. The choices that are left are the ones with the best chance of being the correct answer. Sometimes, by doing it this way, the answer will suddenly come to you as you remember the details. Sometimes you will be down to the last two choices which give you a 50-50 chance of being correct.■

CHAPTER 20
GUIDE TO PERIODIC ASSESSMENT

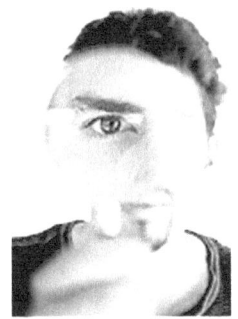

Importance of Periodic Assessments

There are so many people who start their prep by reading through all the study materials. After three months of studying they move on to online q banks and is aghast at how poorly they scored. Then they go into panic mode when they realize they wasted 3 months of prep time and their scheduled exam date is drawing ever nearer. They could have avoided all this by assessing their performance right from the start of their review.

People think that assessment should only be done to see if they are ready to sit for the exam. Although that is important, it is not enough for them to do well in this exam. There seem to be a presumption that they are actually studying effectively from the beginning. Nothing is further from the truth. There is a need to start periodic assessment right from the start of the prep, to assess the effectiveness of their study methods. It is a waste of time to study for 3 whole months only to realize that it was ineffective and little progress has been made.

The prep course is designed so that you do your periodic assessment right from the start of the course. This way any problems in your study methods that will impact your progress can be identified early on and remedial measures implemented right away. This ensures effective review right from the start and ensures that you don't waste any time.

How to Do Periodic Assessments during Review

When you talk assessment, most people think either of the NBME assessment tests or the online q banks. In reality, there are different types of assessment you need to do throughout your review and it's best to use different types of tests to do so.

The first assessment you should do is to test the effectiveness of your study methods. It is important to ensure that you are prepping the right way from the very start. Otherwise, you would have wasted a lot of time prepping ineffectively with little or no progress. In the course, you start your prep with per chapter quizzes you take immediately after finishing each chapter. This insures that you need to have learned or retained enough information of the chapter before you move on to the next one. It also means that in case there is a problem in your study methods, it is resolved early enough in your prep to impact your review positively. It's best to use quiz books that mirror the chapters you study in the course. For Pathology, we use Robbin's Review of Pathology and an online quiz in the prep site. For Microbiology and Immunology, we use Levinson and Jawetz, Review of Microbiology and Immunology. The end of the book has a series of quiz that covers each section of Microbiology and Immunology.

For Pharmacology, we use Trevor and Katzung's Pharmacology Review for our per chapter quiz. There is no recommended per chapter quiz for the minor four. It is expected that by the time you finish the big three, you would have corrected any errors in your study methods already. Plus, doing per chapter quiz is very effective but also very time-consuming. The extra review time is worth the effort for the big three, since they occupy such a big percentage of USMLE Step 1, but not for the minor 4.

The next type of assessment is to assess whether you are progressing through the prep properly. First, are you integrating the topics between subjects properly? Then, are you integrating topics between subjects correctly. This can usually be assessed by various question books and online q banks. For within subject integration, using Kaplan's Q Book which presents question by subject tests your integration of topics within subject. Online Q banks and other integrated q bank like Rapid Review are good for testing your integration between subjects.

Next you need to assess your ability to read fast and recall fast. You can use flashcards and various q banks for that. In the course, we use online flashcards made specifically for improving and assessing your ability to recall the information. We also use q banks with very short direct to the point questions, to improve fast recall. Flashcards can be used for all subjects but are most effective for subjects that require you to memorize lots of different topics that are unrelated to each other like anatomy, microbiology and pharmacology. For subjects that are mostly processes, the best type of flashcards to use are illustrations and algorithms. This includes physiology and biochemistry.

If you are doing 3 revisions as recommended in this course, you would have studied all the subjects and integrated the subjects together. There is a need to assess for weak points in your review. Even if you have already studied all the topics in detail, you will still have weak points. The reason is that we have different interests and we pay more attention to topics we are interested in. So even if you have read everything, your mind would have paid less attention to subjects you are not interested in. You may have been reading the words, but your mind wanders off. Therefore those topics will be your weak points. But the USMLE tests what it thinks you need to know in order to practice medicine in the United States. It does not care whether you are interested in the topic or not. If its important it will come out. Therefore, you need to cover your weak points. This is usually done when you are doing the online Q banks like Kaplan and USMLE World.

Lastly, you need to assess your readiness for sitting for the exam. The correct assessment tools to use for this are the NBME online assessment tests. Some people prefer to use the UW assessment tests, but per experience, the NBME tests are more predictive and consistent while the UW assessment tests tend to overestimate your predicted score. With these excellent tools available for you to insure that you are ready to take the exam and give you more or less a good estimate of how you will perform, it is a wonder people still sit for the exam without taking this assessment tests and failing in the process.

If you notice, I do not advocate you take a pre-test to assess your weak and strong points at the start of the course. The main reason is that for most people, prior to starting a formal prep, everything is a weak point. Only when you are making a final high yield review do you need to focus on correcting weak points. Plus the USMLE does not give the same weight to all the different subjects and therefore it is best to concentrate on subjects that carry the most weight. Only after insuring you are very strong on the big three, do you start concentrating on the minor four.■

CHAPTER 21

MASTERING CLINICAL VIGNETTES

Importance of Clinical Vignettes

With the clinical slant of the USMLE, clinical vignettes have become increasingly important and more questions are in the form of clinical cases. We need to understand that the mandate of the USMLE is to test for the medical students' readiness to practice clinical medicine in the US. Hence, it is important for the medical student to know how to apply the principles of basic medical science in clinical practice.

Whenever the questions are in the form of clinical vignettes, you need to make a diagnosis first before you even have a chance at answering the question. Questions in the USMLE usually center on a particular topic about a particular disease. You need to know what particular disease you are dealing with before you know what you need to answer about that particular disease. On average people lose 2 to 3 questions per block due to inability to diagnose the case. In other words, if they had been able to diagnose the case, then they would have gotten the answer. So if you are missing less than that, then your ability to diagnose clinical vignettes is very good. If you are missing more than that, then you need to work on your ability to diagnose clinical vignettes.

Classical and Atypical Presentation of Clinical Cases

The cases you meet in clinical practice can be divided into common or rare cases and their presentations into classical and atypical presentations. The cases you meet in order of frequency are first, common cases with classical presentations. Then common cases with atypical presentations. Followed by rare cases with classical presentations and lastly rare cases with atypical presentation.

In Step 1, the cases you encounter will mostly have classical presentations, although you will encounter both common and rare cases. The main deciding factor on what cases appear in Step 1 is whether they illustrate a basic principle in basic medical science. For example, both Prader-Willi and Angelman Syndrome are very rare, but they illustrate the genetic principle of imprinting. Therefore, you can expect this rare case to appear in Step 1, even though you may never get to see it in real life.

In Step 2 CK and Step 3 on the other hand, most of the cases you will meet are of the common types. However, be prepared to meet some atypical presentations. Don't be surprised if cases contain irrelevant positive and negative findings. There is a saying in clinical medicine that if you hear the pounding of hooves, it usually is best to think of horses, but be prepared that sometimes, it could be zebras. Also true for the USMLE.

How to Train Yourself to Diagnose Clinical Vignettes

From the very start, you should pay attention to the typical signs and symptoms associated with each disease. In Step 1 Review, you encounter this when you study Pathology, therefore do not ignore them and take time to study them well. It also makes sense to correlate the particular signs or symptoms as they relate to the pathology itself. The signs and symptoms are either due to disruption of the anatomic structure or underlying physiologic or biochemical processes, or caused by the body's response to these disruptions either in an attempt to compensate or restore function. Understanding how these symptoms and signs relate to the underlying pathologic process can help you understand and remember them more thoroughly.

A good example is relating the various heart sounds and murmurs to various pathology of the heart. We know that the first and second heart sounds are produced by valvular movements. Understanding how these valvular movements change with pathology and how the corresponding heart sound changes can make it easier to understand the symptoms that accompany that pathology.

Another example is breath sounds. Most people will associate wheezing with asthma. But knowing that wheezing is caused by narrowing of mid-sized bronchi means other pathology can cause wheezing too and must be ruled out.

However, the above is just the start. Studying signs and symptoms this way is not enough for you to be able to diagnose cases. The reason is that diagnosing cases require your thinking process be the reverse. When you study the disease, you typically start with the disease and then you memorize the signs and symptoms. In diagnosis, it's the reverse, you start with signs and symptoms, and then you try to diagnosis what disease the patient have. Studying them the first way, with disease first will not make it easy for you to diagnose cases with symptoms first.

Also, in medical school, you were taught to use differential diagnosis in order to diagnose a case. But it's not a good idea to depend on differential diagnosis in the USMLE, namely because of time constraint. Considering every possible diagnosis one at a time takes too much time, which you don't have in the USMLE. Plus most experienced clinicians do not use differential diagnosis as the primary means of arriving at a diagnosis. They use pattern recognition. Each disease has a pattern of presentation. And identifying this pattern, you arrive at a diagnosis. Don't get me wrong, in more complicated cases;

we still do differential diagnosis to supplement this pattern recognition. So too in the exam, you need to use pattern recognition to diagnose cases, reserving differential diagnosis for tougher cases, else you won't finish the exam because you will run out of time.

If you are having problems with clinical vignettes, one of the things you can do is either get the book Pretest Physical Diagnosis or sign up online for the High Yield Clinical Vignette course on my prep site or both. Pretest is composed of 500 questions of which about 300++ deals with classical presentation of diseases. The diagnosis is usually on one of the choices. You start by reading the question and choose the diagnosis from the list. Once you can do that very well, try to diagnose the case without looking thru the choices. That will train you to recognize classic cases without having the answer choices as clues, which is usually the case in the actual exam.

If you decide to enrol on the High Yield Clinical Vignette course in my prep site, instructions on how to use that is on the site.■

CHAPTER 22
SPEED READING

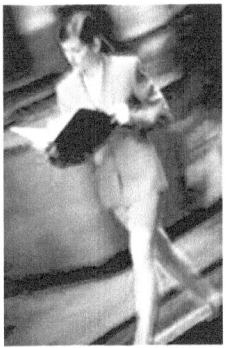

Why You Need to Read Fast

There are two main reasons why you need to be able to read fast for the USMLE.

First, you are required to read, understand and memorize huge amount of materials. Being able to read fast will help you cover more grounds faster. Understand also, that the more materials you are able to read, understand and memorize, the higher your score will be. So reading fast can help push your score up.

Second, USMLE questions tend to be long. In fact some questions can be described as kilometric or especially long. Since the USMLE is a time-pressured exam, being able to read fast can help you finish questions faster and thus help you get a higher score.

How We Read

When we first learn to read, we had to learn abc's first. Then we learn that stringing the alphabet together produces words. Stringing words together produces phrases and sentences. Putting together sentences produces a paragraph and multiple paragraphs form a section or a chapter. And we also realize central to each of this unit of writing is one idea.

When we started reading, we were taught to read out loud. The reason for reading out loud is so that our teachers can know whether we are reading correctly or not. As we grow older, we take this habit with us and we tend to vocalize or subvocalize what we read. Some people still read the words under their breath or form the words with their mouth. Those who subvocalize either say it silently on their throat, or say it in their minds enunciating each word. These are usually the slowest readers going less than a hundred words per minute.

Some people start realizing that they don't have to read every word in order to understand what is written. They realized that if they read in phrases they can still understand what the material is talking about. It's not long before they start skipping prepositions, conjunctions, etc. as well. Even if they skip the: and, the, a, an, is, to, in etc., they realize that their mind will automatically fill in the missing word. Once they start doing this, they realize they can actually read much faster, about 50 to 100% faster than before.

But you can actually go much faster than that. One of the things that limit how fast we can go is the need to subvocalize words. If you need to read it out loud, you will go really slowly. If you just need to form the words with your lips you will go that much faster. If you subvocalize, i.e. hear the sound with your mind but not aloud, you can go even faster. When you subvocalize this way, you actually make very soft sounds in your vocal cord which can be picked up by sensitive equipment.

When you stop subvocalizing completely, then you can start reading with your mind. There are two ways you can do these. First you still 'read' the words, but you are moving so fast since you are not limited by the speed of your vocal cords but how fast your eyes can move through the words. You can go through books very fast, reaching speeds close to a thousand words per minute. But to read really, really fast, you have to learn how to read pages like you read photographs.

When you look at a photograph, you don't have to look at every aspect of a photograph in order to know what a photograph is all about. Your brain takes in a whole photograph, processes it and presents the result of the process to your brain for interpretation. In reality, your brain has the capacity to look at a written page and do the same. And there are people who can do that. The reason you and I can't do it is because we were not trained to 'read' that way. We were trained to read word for word and the reason was that so our teachers know that we 'know' how to read those words. But with proper training, what can be achieved is short of miraculous. That is how people can read thousands of words per minute. Finish a large book in a few minutes and tell you what it's all about. Because they are now reading at the speed of thought!!

However, you need to be trained this way while still a child. If you read the section on How we learn under Learning Phase Basics, you will understand why it's hard to learn something new as we grow older. In my case I started learning speed reading in my teens. So I never reached the ability to read in pages or paragraphs. I can read in sentences but not always. My fastest speed is about 1000 words per minute or thereabouts. That's about 2.5 to 3 pages of a pocketbook per minute. If you are now in your 20's, you can still improve your reading speed from 20 to 50%.

One thing critics decry about speed reading is the fact that a speed reader cannot always detect a wrongly spelled word or poor grammar. What this shows is that the critic does not understand what speed reading is all about. The reason you can read that fast is that you don't read word for word. You depend on your brain to fill in the blank and get the gist of what you are reading. Therefore, you can't really detect a misspelled word, because your brain will correct it when it interprets it. That's why you can't speed read when you are proof reading something, because you need to look at every word in order to edit them.

Another problem with speed reading is that although you get the meaning of what you are reading, part of the pleasure of reading is the play on words the author use. Hence the popularity of collecting quotes. So you sometimes have to read slowly to savor the taste of the flow of words. Speed reading gives you the option to change how fast you read depending on the situation. It's like having a car. If you need to get somewhere fast you can. But once in a while you need to drive slow to enjoy the scenery better. So too with speed reading.

How to Speed Read

So how do you learn to speed read? We are presuming you are an adult of course and therefore, it's not really that easy to double or triple your reading speed. Plus you have a few months to prep for the USMLE not a few years, so the best we can probably hope for is to improve your reading speed by 20 to 30%. So how do we start?

First, we need to establish how you read right now. Do you read word for word? Do you move your mouth when you read? Do you subvocalize? The first step is to stop doing that. Try to read by phrase. Drop the: *a, an, the, to,* etc. at this point you would still be subvocalizing, but you won't be reading every word and that will speed you up. You may be uncomfortable at first. You feel that you may be missing something. But when you try to explain what you have read, you will find out that you didn't miss much. After a few weeks, you will find it comfortable reading this way and you will be reading much, much faster.

So, you are now reading by phrase and not word for word, however, you are still subvocalizing. How do we reduce subvocalizing or eliminate it altogether? The key to getting rid of sub vocalization is to go through the words so fast you don't have time to subvocalize. Actually, you can read as fast as your eyes can go through the words and that is several times faster than when you sub vocalize the words.

So how do we make our eyes go through the words faster? --by using your index finger. You use your index finger, underlining the words you are reading. Now make your index finger go faster and follow your fingers. Initially, the words may blur and you have a hard time making out the words. But eventually you will notice that the words will sort of leap out at you. It's your brain processing out the key words that are important for you to understand what you are reading. When this happens, it's time for you to move your fingers even faster and you will read faster. It will take a few weeks before you get used to this type of reading, but you will notice that you are now reading very fast with very little lost of comprehension. If you notice you are having a hard time comprehending a particular part of what you are reading, slow down a bit and then speed back up on the easy parts. Using the car analogy, when negotiating rougher parts of the roads or sharp bends, you need to slow down a bit, but on good roads, you can throttle the engine and breeze right through.

Using the above methods, you can read phrases at a time or even sentences at a time. But how do you get to read paragraphs or even pages at a time? Again with the help of your magic index finger. However, unless you are very young, around pre-teens, you might have a hard time getting used to reading this way. I couldn't since I started when I was in my teens. But I know someone who started at age 7 and he has no problem reading this way. Anyway, I will describe the method for those interested in knowing the detail.

The goal is to make sure your eye goes through all the words in the paragraph. You place your finger on the first word of the paragraph and move along the line, but instead of moving to the second line, you move your finger across the paragraph to the left lower corner of the paragraph. You then move across the last line of the paragraph, then move your finger across the paragraph to the left upper corner where you began. Forming an X. This will train your eyes to start looking at the paragraph as a whole rather than individual words or sentences. Reading pages uses the same principle. You do the same thing but for whole pages rather than paragraphs. Again, this is for young kids only, older people will have a really tough time learning to read this way.■

CHAPTER 23
IMPROVING RECALL

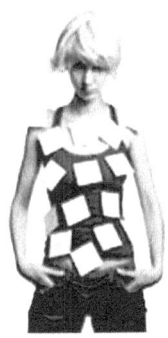

Importance of Recall in the USMLE

For the purpose of the USMLE, what you cannot recall, usually in a minute or less, you do not know. The USMLE does not really care whether you know or have memorized something, unless you can recall it during the exam itself, you get no credit or even partial points. A lot of times the reason you can't answer the question is not because you do not know the topic, or have not memorized it. The most common reason is that you can't recall it fast enough for the exam. Many times people recall the answer only after they walk out of the exam room and as I said, the USMLE don't even give them partial points for that.

Since the USMLE will give you credit only for things you can recall, the only thing that really counts in the exam is your ability to recall the information you have memorized. So even if you did everything else, read every material available, spend hours memorizing, burning the midnight oil, gone through thousands of questions through the q banks, if you cannot recall the information fast enough to answer the question during the exam, you get no points. Therefore, it seems only logical that you spend as much time as possible improving your ability to recall what you have studied and memorize and make sure you can recall them fast enough for the exam. And yet you would be surprised how little attention most people put on improving their ability to recall information for the USMLE.

So, how do I improve retention and recall? First we will discuss basic principles on how we retain and recall information. Then we will discuss specific methods of improving retention and recall of information.

Three R's of Retention and Recall

How we retain and recall information is rooted on how we learn. Please read details on How We Learn on the appropriate section. In short, our brain forms synapse between neurons every time we learn something. The more often we make use of the synapse, i.e. try to recall or encounter the same information, the stronger the connection the more we remember. The less we recall or encounter that information, the connection weakens and we tend to forget. This weakening is a function of time.

These basic principles bring us to the three R's of retention and recall, namely, Repetition, Relation and Recency. We need to take advantage of the three R's in our prep in order to maximize our retention and recall of what we have learned.

Repetition is the most important principle in memorizing anything. In fact whenever a student tells me that he is having a hard time memorizing, my suggestion is that repeat it often enough and you will remember it. It is memorization by brute force. The main problem with repetition is that it is a very time consuming process. Relying on repetition alone to memorize, retain and recall information will take a long time. As kids a lot of times we memorize using sheer repetition. Everybody remembers the countless repetitions of our ABC's and the multiplication table as some examples. However, as adults, our ability to memorize and recall information by sheer repetition is not as powerful as when we were kids. This has to do with the maturation of our CNS and therefore we have to rely on other principles to make memorizing, retaining and recalling information better.

Relation is the best way for adults to memorize things. Relating something to what one already knows makes it easier to remember it. The more linkages you have to a particular concept the stronger your ability to retain and recall that concept. Therefore it is important to create as many linkages as you can between concepts. That's part of the reason that throughout the course you are encouraged to integrate everything you study and study concepts from different context for better retention.

Recency is the third principle of retention and recall. The more recently you recall or encounter any information, the stronger your retention of it. Forgetting is a function of time. In the course, we take advantage of this principle by doing multiple revisions and having a high yield review just before sitting for the exam. This insures that you remember most strongly concepts that have the highest chance of coming out in the exam.

Specific Methods to Improve Retention and Recall

Knowing the three R's of Retention and Recall, it is important for us to apply these principles throughout our prep. Askdoc's USMLE Step 1 Prep Course is designed to take advantage of these principles in order to maximize your ability to do well in this exam.

First, we do at least three revisions in the course. Doing

multiple revisions take advantage of the principle of repetition. In reality, the more revisions you do the higher your score will go but only up to a certain point. Because we do burn out and plateau eventually.

Doing multiple revisions also try to take advantage of the principle of recency. The USMLE is such a huge undertaking that by the time you finish one revision, so much time would have passed that you would have forgotten a big chunk of what you studied at the start. But subsequent revisions, take less time to finish and by the third revision the time interval is short enough that you have forgotten very little of it.

Second, you are asked to integrate both within a subject and between subjects. Integration and correlation take advantage of two principles of retention, namely repetition and relation. When you integrate topics, you need to read them at least twice. Once to understand the topic, second to relate them to another topic. It also takes advantage of the principle of relation. As you integrate topics together, you relate them to other topics you already know. These relations reinforce each other, making it easier for you to recall all of them.

Third, you are asked to organize topics into headings and subheadings, memorize them and link everything else you studied to these headings and subheadings. This step creates an organized framework to relate things to each other and remember them much more easily. In fact, you are even asked to create a framework primarily for Pathology and instead of creating a separate framework for anatomy and physiology to just relate them into Pathology so as to strengthen the relation.

Fourth, by using the principles on how to memorize list of items and studying processes, we again take advantage of the principles of repetition and relation. Knowing the difference between things relates them together as much as knowing what is similar about them. By doing step by step comparison, we also do a lot of repetition. Both steps increase our ability to remember and retain the information studied that way.

Fifth, we stressed the need to study the concepts under different context. Again this makes use of two principles, namely relation and repetition.

Lastly, we put in a high yield review in the end. Mainly to take advantage of the principles of repetition and recency to make sure we remember the concepts most tested in the exam.

Specific Methods of Improving Recall

There are also some methods we employ to improve recall primarily. One of the ways you can do this is that after finishing a chapter or a section of a chapter, you try to recite out loud what you have read without looking at your notes. In fact, a good way of doing this is to explain what you have just read to someone else. Another way is to illustrate it like a diagram on a board or list down the main points and recite out loud the details.

One of the reasons you do per chapter quiz for the big three is to practice and test how well you have recalled what you have memorized. Recalling something immediately after you have tried to memorize it is a good way to improve your retention and ability to recall that information.

Another method we employ is with the use of flashcards. In order for flashcards to help you recall information very fast, each flashcards must contain only one specific topic or concept. Most commercial flashcards cram too much topic under one card. So you are better off making your own.

Starting on your second revision, we also employ a speed building q bank to help you recall things faster and randomly. Since we tend to study information in groups and relate them to each other, it is easier for us to recall information in the order we organize them. However, a lot of times, you have to recall things randomly in the USMLE and it pays to practice random recall. ■

CHAPTER 24
HOW TO INTEGRATE WITHIN SUBJECT

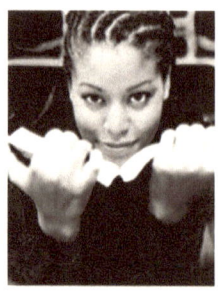

Integrating within a Subject

Medicine is such a large discipline that it is impossible to learn everything all at once. Hence there is a need to divide them into subjects. But even each subject is rather large and most books on these subjects divide the topics into even smaller pieces into chapters. Each chapter is then divided into smaller sections or subtopics of the chapters.

Studying topics in small pieces may make it easier to understand, but there is a danger of being unable to see the subject as a whole. That is missing the forest for the trees. USMLE will test both your understanding of each subject as a whole as well as details of individual topics. Therefore it is important to integrate the different topics and chapters to each other so as to understand the subject as a whole. For more detailed discussions of each subject and how to do within subject integration, refer to the discussions on how to review individual subjects.

Integrating Anatomy

Anatomy is composed of four sub disciplines, which means we have to do a lot of integration among its sub disciplines, namely Gross Anatomy, Neuroanatomy, Histology and Embryology.

Gross Anatomy is the big daddy of Anatomy, in terms of total amount of subject matter you need to cover in Anatomy it's around 50%. There are usually two ways gross anatomy is presented, by region and by systems. You need to study them both ways. Studying them by region is more important for Surgery, but studying by systems makes more sense for pathophysiology and understanding mechanisms of disease. Therefore you need to integrate them both ways and be able to switch your thinking either way.

Neuroanatomy is a very important sub discipline in anatomy. You need to understand not only neural pathways, but their blood supply, relationship with surrounding anatomic structures and syndromes or deficits associated with pathology located in all three. You need to know them in an integrated way and not piecemeal.

Histology can be referred to as microscopic anatomy. You need to be able to integrate the microscopic structure of the cells and tissues to the corresponding anatomic structure. For example, cell structure of the lining of the alveoli is unique to the respiratory system. It is optimized for gas exchange between the environment and the human body.

Embryology is also known as developmental anatomy. You need to correlate development of the anatomic structure from embryologic origins to its adult state.

Integrating Physiology

Physiology is always divided by systems as it is easier to understand it that way. However, we need to understand that these systems do interact. Therefore, we need to integrate the various systems together in order to truly understand physiology. For example, blood pressure is basically controlled by four different systems. The cardiovascular system, i.e. heart and blood vessels, the nervous system, i.e. vagus nerve, sympathetic, parasympathetic neurons, endocrine, i.e. adrenals, renin-angiotensin system and renal system, i.e. kidney. So you need to integrate the topics together to fully understand blood pressure control.

Integrating Biochemistry

Biochemistry deals with two subjects primarily. Metabolism and Genetics. For metabolism it is important to understand the metabolism of each substrate and how these substrates and products of these substrates affect its own metabolism. These substrates also affect the metabolism of other substrates and understanding how this happens is crucial to understanding metabolism as a whole. The metabolism of proteins, carbohydrates and fats are interrelated with common pathways and other interactions that require integration.

Genetics, although covered mainly in biochemistry is an integrated topics. Molecular biology is encountered in various disciplines like cell biology, cell physiology and pathology. Therefore, it is important to understand that to understand genetics, you need to integrate a lot of topics.

Integrating Pathology

Pathology is a subject that tries to integrate what you know of anatomy, physiology and biochemistry into explaining the pathology of diseases. It requires a lot of reading and analysis in order to master the topics. But the subject itself is mainly divided into two parts, general pathology and systems pathology.

General pathology covers general pathologic mechanisms that apply to most systems while systems pathology discusses specific pathologic mechanisms applicable to individual systems. You need to integrate these specific pathologic processes to the general process that occurs in all systems. For example, general process of necrosis and cell death occurs in all cells of all systems. However, depending on the system involve, the exact pathologic mechanisms will differ and those differences are very important because they will be tested by the USMLE. Although the pathology of neoplasia for different systems is generally similar, there are enough differences that you need to take note of.

Another thing you need to integrate are pathologic diseases that occur across systems. For example hypertension usually affects multiple systems in the body and some hormonal problems can cause other hormonal problems, i.e. hypothyroidism causing hyperprolactinemia, etc. A lot of times, the discussions even in textbooks end by just pointing towards what needs to be integrated. You still need to go through the details and integrate them yourself.

Integrating Pharmacology

Integrating Pharmacology involves knowing how to differentiate drugs that belong to different subclasses. For example diuretics are divided into different subclasses like osmotic diuretics, thiazides, loop diuretics, potassium-sparing diuretics and ADH antagonist. You not only need to know the details of each drug, you need to be able to differentiate them from each other. Another important step you need to do is differentiate the drugs within a subclass. This usually involves knowing the prototype for each subclass and understanding the differences between the major variant drugs of that subclass vs. the prototype drugs.

Integrating Microbiology and Immunology

Microbiology is divided into Basic and Clinical Bacteriology, Basic and Clinical Virology, Mycology and Parasitology. Most of the integration you need to do is between Basic and Clincial Bacteriology and between Basic and

Mike Nicol Uy, MD

Clinical Virology. Basic Bacteriology discusses general characteristics of bacterial organisms while Clinical Bacteriology discusses specific characteristics of individual bacterial organisms. You need to correlate those general and specific characteristics and understand what is the same and what is different. Same thing holds true for Basic and Clinical Virology. ∎

CHAPTER 25
HOW TO INTEGRATE BETWEEN SUBJECTS

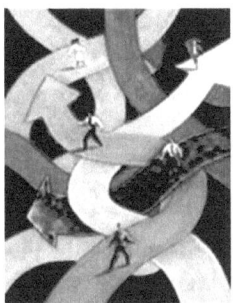

Integrating Between Subjects

One of the most important things you need to do in order to do well in Step 1 is to integrate the different topics in the different subjects together. The more integration you have done, the better you understand the basic sciences. The better you understand the basic sciences, the higher score you get. One of the big reasons why Goljan's pathology lectures and notes are so effective in raising scores is that it covers a lot of integrated topic. Even then, Goljan does not cover every topic that needs to be integrated.

One of the big reasons why reading Robbin's Pathologic Basis of Disease can raise scores a lot is that it does a lot of integration between subjects in the discussions. The problem of course lies in the size of the text and not everyone can invest the time reading it. So most settle for Goljan's pathology lectures and notes. Even Robbin's misses a crucial integration which is tested in the USMLE. It does not integrate Pathology and Pharmacology. You probably need Harrison's or Cecil's Textbook of Medicine, but even they do not really discuss them in detail.

So the best way to really do integration is doing it yourself rather than depend on these books to do it for you, although they can help. Of course you have to know how to integrate topics in the first place and this is the purpose of this chapter.

We need to understand that all pathology starts as disruption of either an anatomic structure or a physiologic or biochemical process or all three. These disruption causes a disequilibrium or even a loss of function and the body attempts to restore function or equilibrium by either repairing the anatomic structure or physiologic or biochemical process that was disrupted or compensating for them. In turn this attempt at compensation and restoration can restore function and equilibrium or cause further disruption until the body reaches a new state of equilibrium or it fails altogether and the patient dies. Therefore, you need to integrate Anatomy, Physiology and Biochemistry into Pathology in order to understand the process as a whole.

All types of therapeutic interventions aims to restore or compensate for the disequilibrium caused by the pathologic process. For Step 1, we only consider one type of therapeutic intervention, pharmacotherapy. The other type of intervention like surgery, radiation, etc is covered in other steps. Therefore, we need to integrate Pharmacology into Pathology, too. We also need to understand that any pharmacologic intervention has the possibility of causing further disruptions and so on and so forth.

Integration means putting all these together so you understand the big picture. Then you need to memorize the details of these integrated topics to be able to recall them in the exam. Actually you can do your integration during the exam proper itself as long as you know the appropriate details. However, integrating topics together can be a long thinking process and you have only on average barely a minute to answer each question in the USMLE. So doing your integration during prep time is highly recommended.

Integrating Anatomy and Physiology

First you need to integrate Anatomy and Physiology. Structure and function correlation helps you understand how the human body works normally. And that is the basis for understanding everything else that follows. For example, the anatomic structure of the lungs and the bony thorax is optimized for air exchange. What salient features account for this efficiency? Even the microscopic structures of the cells and tissues of the respiratory tract is optimized for gas exchange. How is this accomplished? Another example is the kidney, the nephron is arranged to optimize the countercurrent mechanisms responsible for concentrating the urine. How does its structure accomplish this? What about the structure of the glomerular apparatus? How does this optimize filtration? The structure of the blood vessels supplying the kidney differs slightly from the rest of the body. How does this difference enhance the function of the kidney?

There is a systematic way of doing this. First, I read about a specific anatomic structure. Then I open my physiology book to the equivalent system. Then I ask the question, how does this specific anatomic structure accomplish its function. By doing that systematically, I usually cover everything that needs to be covered.

Integrating Biochemistry into Anatomy and Physiology

Biochemical reactions need to be integrated into appropriate sections of anatomy and physiology. Most biochemical processes occur in the cellular level, therefore it is important to integrate with appropriate topics in cell biology(a subtopic of histology). Metabolism of substrate occurs on various organs and systems of the body and should be integrated into the appropriate topics in anatomy and physiology. Genetics is also very important. Molecular genetics are the basis for many pathologic diseases and understanding how they normally control the human body's development and function is crucial to understanding pathophysiology.

Integrating Pathology to the Minor Three

It is recommended that you use pathology to organize your integration. When it comes time to memorize the integrated topics, use pathology as the main subject, integrating the minor three, anatomy, physiology and biochemistry into topics in pathology. One good thing about pathology, especially textbooks like Robbin's is that they incorporate some discussions on integration, especially the minor three. The main problem is that the discussions do not go deep enough into the minor three, so relying on pathology texts alone for integration will limit the total benefit you will gain by integrating between subjects.

Whenever you are integrating pathology, always ask yourself, what anatomic structure, or physiologic or biochemical process is disrupted. What does the anatomic structure look like or do or how does the physiologic or biochemical process normally function? What equilibrium does it maintain in the body? How does the pathology cause disruption or loss of function? What disequilibrium happens? How does the body respond to this disequilibrium short term? Long term? What compensation mechanism happens? What reparative process happens? Does these compensation or reparative process cause other pathology?

When you depend on pathology books to do some of the integration for you, you come up with a problem. Although they usually discuss the pathology thoroughly, they discuss relevant topics in anatomy, physiology and biochemistry superficially. So if you have to, go to the relevant topic in any of the three subjects and cover them thoroughly. Don't make the presumption as a lot of people do that since you read the three subjects a few months before, or that you are going to read it one to two months later, that your mind will automatically integrate the details for you. If you do that, you will find that during the exam, you can't remember the detailed integration at all. And if you start the thought process of integrating it during the exam proper itself, you run out of time before you reach the answer. So do the full integration during review not during the exam where you have very limited time.

Integrating Physiology and Biochemistry into Pharmacology

Understanding Pharmacology properly requires you to integrate them with relevant topics in physiology and biochemistry. It is fairly obvious that all drugs act on either a physiologic or biochemical process in the body. A good way to integrate this is to start with a physiologic or biochemical process. Then fill in where the drugs act on the process. It is even better of you can divide the drugs into those that enhance the process, those that slow down or stop the process or those that modify the process. It actually makes it easier to understand where the drugs work and how they work.

Integrating Pathology into Pharmacology

Now that you understand how pathology occurs and you understand how drugs basically affect processes, you now need to integrate pathology to pharmacology. Remember that pathology involves disruption of processes and the compensatory and reparative actions of the body. To help the body compensate and restore function and equilibrium, we use drugs. And the action of these drugs is on the physiologic and biochemical processes themselves. We also need to be aware that drugs themselves can cause disruption of other processes. This disruption of other processes or what we consider side effects or adverse reaction can by themselves cause further pathology. You need to integrate these topics as far as you can.

Integrating Pathology and Pharmacology into Physiology and Biochemistry

Instead of doing just a limited integration of pathology and pharmacology, you can opt to do a full cycle integration of both subjects directly with physiology and biochemistry. It is more complicated integration process than just simply integrating pathology to pharmacology, but it gives you a more thorough picture of the integrated topic. This is the way I actually did it in my own prep.

You start with a physiologic or biochemical process. Try to fill in where specific pathology disrupts specific steps of the process. Understand how these disruptions affect the process as a whole. Then you add in where the drugs act in specific steps of the process. Ask yourself whether the drugs act at the point of pathology in the process or before or after it. Determine how these correct the pathology, aggravates it, or even cause pathology somewhere else.

Microbiology and Immunology - an Integrated Subject

Microbiology and Immunology is actually a good example of integrated topics. It puts together topics in physiology, biochemistry, pathology and pharmacology in a single discussion but focused on infectious diseases. Ideally that should be how integrated your knowledge of all other pathology is. If you can do that for all other diseases, then you are probably on your way to a high score.■

***

unit 4

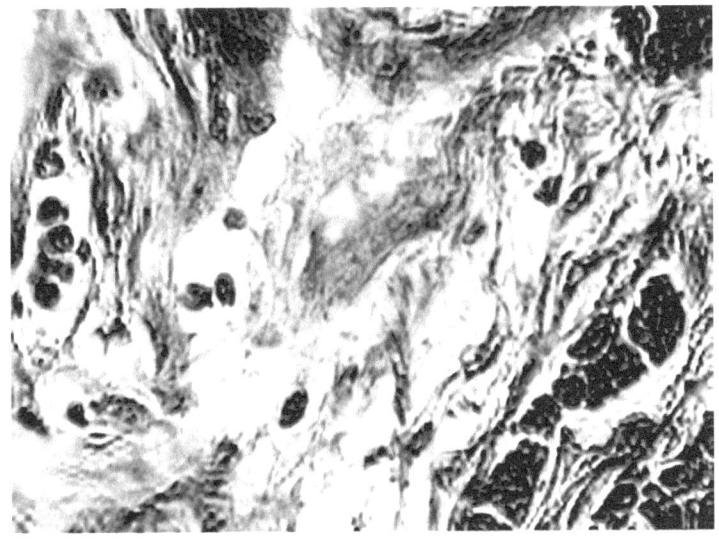

How to Review Pathology

CHAPTER 26
INTRODUCTION

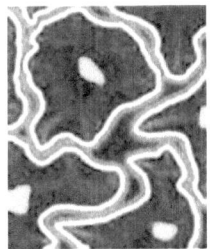

Pathology is the Most Important Subject in Step 1

The purpose of Step 1 is to test your knowledge of basic medical science as it applies to clinical practice. Core to that knowledge is a basic understanding of not only the normal anatomic structure and physiologic and biochemical processes, but how disease can alter normal structure and processes. Understanding of how pathology happens is crucial in understanding how to treat them.

So we should not be surprised why pathology is the most important subject in Step 1. In fact a substantial percentage of Step 2 CK and Step 3 also cover pathology. Some of the toughest questions you will encounter in the USMLE will be pathology questions. The level of detail you need to know in pathology in order to be able to answer those questions is also substantial.

Pathology is the Biggest Subject with Lots of Details

Aside from being the biggest subject in terms of content among all the 7 subjects covered in the USMLE Step 1, it also covers the biggest percentage in terms of questions that will come out in the exam. Therefore, pathology can be considered the most high-yield of all the subjects in Step 1. However, be aware that more than any other subject, the level of detail in pathology is tremendous and you need to master a lot of them.

Pathology Integrates Knowledge in Anatomy, Physiology and Biochemistry

In order to understand pathology fully, you need to integrate knowledge in anatomy, physiology and biochemistry. Without a deeper understanding of the 3 more basic subjects, it's a lot harder to memorize pathology. Therefore when you review pathology properly, you are forced to review the 3 other subjects, too. Therefore, studying pathology well can help you actually perform better in all these subjects.■

CHAPTER 27

STUDY MATERIALS FOR PATHOLOGY

Study materials for pathology can be divided into *texts, reviewers, flashcards and q banks.*

Textbooks include the following
- Robbin's Pathologic Basis of Diseases
- Robbin's Basic Pathology

Reviewers include
- Askdoc's Pathology Notes - Study Notes, Outline Notes, Summary Notes
- Kaplan's Lecture Notes - Section on Pathology
- BRS Pathology
- NMS Pathology
- Goljan's Rapid Review of Pathology
- Goljan's Audio Lecture and Notes
- First Aid - Section on Pathology

Flashcards include
- Askdoc's High Yield Flashcards for Pathology
- BRS Flashcards for Pathology

Q banks include
- Robbin's Review of Pathology
- Rapid Review for Pathology Q bank
- Kaplan's Q Book - Section on Pathology
- Kaplan's Online Q Bank - Section on Pathology
- USMLE World Online Q Bank - Section on Pathology

We will discuss the more important study materials in

more detail.

Askdoc's Pathology Notes - Study Notes, Outline Notes, Summary Notes

Askdoc's Pathology Notes are the recommended study material for the course. The notes follow all the study methodologies and principles of learning taught in the course. The Study Notes cover all the topics that will be tested in the exam. It covers both low yield and high yield topics. The outline notes cover the high yield topics for high yield review. The summary notes contain instructions and explanations on how to study each chapter properly.

BRS Pathology

This book is probably one of the best high yield review book for Pathology. It covers the right concepts emphasized in the boards. Its main weak point is lack of discussions in pathophysiology. However, since its primary focus is high yield, it presumes you already know them and just need a quick review to remember them. This is slightly larger than my outline notes for Pathology. It is not recommended that you use it alone in your prep unless you are already solidly grounded in Pathology and Pathophysiology and just need a quick review.

NMS Pathology

This book gives fair coverage to both pathology and pathophysiology. However, with all the excellent books on pathology available, it's just not worth your time and money to use this book.

Kaplan Lecture Notes on Pathology

This book has good coverage and gives a solid review. Having said that, there are a lot of better books out there. Goljan's cover pathophysiology better. BRS Pathology is better at covering topics emphasized in the board. Use only if other alternatives are not available.

Robbin's Pathologic Basis of Diseases

If there is one book that can help you get a really high score in the USMLE Step 1, it is this book. However, the problem is it's a very big book, covers both high yield and low yield stuff and not everyone can read through this book and get the maximum benefit. You need to be able to read fast, have a very good memory and can pick out the high yield stuff and discard what won't come out in the exam. If you can do that, then going through Robbin's is the single best thing you can do to up your score. But if you can't, then you are better off using the other reviewers. Trying to memorize Robbin's when you are not really capable of doing so will not only get you nowhere, but can even burn you out fast.

If you are going for a 99 or >230 then this book is indispensable. It has very good discussions on pathophysiology of most of the diseases. Although reading it at least 2 x is most effective, it's such a big book that it is impractical for most people. Better to take down notes while reading, so you can use the notes for subsequent review. If you are using my online notes, write any additional notes on the margins to supplement my notes.

Another very important reason for reading this book is it covers a lot of Molecular Biology topics.

Robbin's Basic Pathology

This is the smaller version of Robbin's Pathologic Basis of Diseases. Hence, the term 'small' Robbins to differentiate it from the bigger version. It has very good discussions in Pathology and Pathophysiology although not as extensive as Big Robbin's. However, for people who feel Big Robbin's is too big, this is a good alternative. Again if you are planning to ace the exam, Big Robbin's is better. This book is barely adequate.

Robbin's Review of Pathology

Review of Pathology is a very good source of questions for Pathology. Most of the questions are written in the USMLE style. Level of difficulty is above average, but compared to the actual USMLE, the questions are actually easier. However, since this q book is for the pathology shelf exam, it covers a lot of lower yield stuff as well as being more detailed, which makes it more difficult overall than the actual Step 1. This q book is the recommended per chapter quiz in the course.

Goljan's Rapid Review of Pathology

The biggest reason you want to use this book is because it discusses a lot of pathophysiology and does a lot of integration between Pathology and the minor 3. If you feel that both big and small Robbin's is too large for you, then this book is a good substitute. It will help you do well, but if you are aiming to ace this exam, then you should think about using Big Robbin's instead.

Goljan's Live Lecture and Pathology Notes

Like Goljan's Rapid Review of Pathology, you can use his lecture and notes to substitute for Big Robbin's. He covers pathophysiology very well. When you hear him in the lecture saying mechanisms, mechanisms, mechanisms, that's pathophysiology. However, it's still inferior to Big Robbin's. If you like lectures more than reading, than this may be the thing for you, but make sure you use his notes, too. Plus if you really want to ace this exam, then Big Robbin's is what you need.

First Aid - Section on Pathology

First Aid for the USMLE Step 1 is only good for high yield review done a week or two before the exam. Otherwise, there is too little information in the book for a comprehensive review of Pathology. You need to do a comprehensive review if you want to do well. More so if you are an IMG. ∎

CHAPTER 28

WHAT TO STUDY IN PATHOLOGY

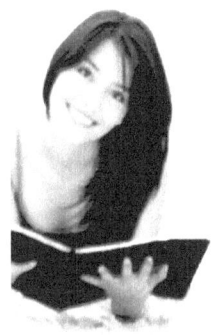

Even though Pathology is the single biggest subject in Step 1, not all the topics in Pathology will come out. There are topics that are more high-yield than others. There are also topics that you need to study in more detail than others. We will give some guidelines on what things are considered more important in pathology. But it is impossible to list everything in detail so you must use your own judgment. An alternative is to use a reviewer like my notes on Pathology. The reviewers reflect what the author thinks is important to study and remember for this exam. It also presents the material at the level of detail the author thinks is appropriate for the exam.

In order to better understand what we need to study we need to understand what the USMLE wants us to know about pathology. Pathology is about diseases and how disease happens. The USMLE wants you to understand how diseases occur in order to understand how to treat it. Therefore, you need to know how diseases happen. You need to understand normal anatomic structure and normal physiologic and biochemical process first. Disruption of these normal structures and processes results in pathology. The study of mechanisms of diseases is called pathophysiology and that is probably where the biggest focus of pathology will be.

The USMLE takes it for granted that you have memorized all the facts. Normal structure, normal processes and the pathologic abnormalities that occurs in diseases. What it wants to know is if you know and understand how normal structures and processes develop pathologic abnormalities and why. Therefore, the most important thing you need to know in pathology is pathophysiology.

With the clinical slant of the USMLE it is important that you be able to diagnose clinical vignettes. This means you need to know the clinical signs and symptoms of diseases. However, in Step 1, the only place you actually encounter descriptions of signs and symptoms of disease is in pathology. Therefore it is important for you to pay particular attention whenever you encounter them.

Pathologic descriptions are the least important especially of the microscopic kind. However, you still need to learn and memorize them. However, unlike pathophysiology, which you have to know like the back of your hand, or the clinical signs and symptoms which you have to know enough to be able to diagnose clinical cases, for pathologic descriptions, know the common ones very well. Be familiar with the less common ones and if you forget a few it's OK. And just ignore the really rare ones.

Pathology is divided into general pathology and systems pathology. In terms of materials you need to memorize, general pathology is about 30% and systems pathology is 70%. But in the exam, about half or a little over half will be about general pathology and systems pathology will around half of pathology. The reason is that general pathology is more important than systems pathology in Step 1. On the other hand, in Step 2 CK and Step 3, the emphasis will be almost entirely on systems pathology.

Lastly, pathologic images and slides. Most of the images and slides in pathology will be the more common and classical ones. Rare diseases and hard to identify images will not be there. That said, most of the images will have descriptions in the question stem that will help you identify what the case is about. So in most cases, there will be enough clues in the question stem to answer the question.

Someone once told me after his exam, that I was wrong and there were a lot of questions with images in which there is not enough clues in the question stem to answer the question. In reality, there was. It's just he did not know enough about the topic tested to be able to answer the question even with the clues. I talked to 4 other people, all high 90's with 1 also a 99 and they all agreed with me that question stems on question with images contain enough clues to answer them even without the images. The guy who said I was wrong got an 82.

CHAPTER 29
FIRST REVISION OF PATHOLOGY

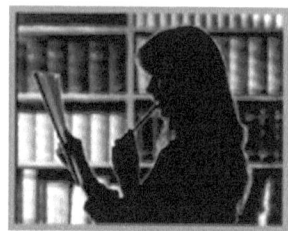

How to Review Pathology

Pathology is the single biggest subject in Step 1. What we call pathology is comprised of pathology and pathophysiology. Pathology deals more with the disease, while pathophysiology deals with how the disease happens or evolves. Most of the integration you need to do is with the pathophysiology portion of pathology rather than pathology. In fact most of the more detailed analysis you need to do during the exam has to do with how disease happens or pathophysiology.

Another thing you have to take note of is the relative importance of general pathology over systems pathology in Step 1. Whereas general pathology is about a third of the typical pathology book or reviewer, it's about half of step 1 pathology. Systems pathology is more important for Step 2 CK and Step 3. It does not mean however that you can ignore systems pathology. It still covers 50% of Step 1 pathology.

Memorize Headings and Subheadings

Pathology is divided into general pathology and systems pathology. General pathology is divided into chapters discussing general pathologic processes like cell pathology, inflammation, neoplasia, etc. Systems pathology is divided into discussions of individual systems and pathologic processes occurring in each of these systems.

Memorizing headings and subheadings is important to provide a general framework and organize what you know and what you are going to learn. Doing it this way makes it easier for you to retain and recall information later.

For example, cell pathology has the following headings: (1) Cell Adaptations to Stress, (2) Causes of Cell Injury, (3) Cellular Changes in Cell Injury, (4) Necrosis, (5) Apoptosis, (6) Intracellular Accumulations. You memorize the headings first. Once you have done that, for each of the headings you go through the subheadings.

For example, subheadings for Intracellular accumulations include the following: (1) Fatty changes, (2) Hyaline changes, (3) Exogenous Pigments, (4) Endogenous Pigments, (5) Pathologic Calcifications.

Memorizing List of Concepts

When memorizing a list of concept, the first step is to memorize all the items on the list. Then you learn to differentiate between the items in the list.

For example, the different types of necrosis include (1) coagulation necrosis, (2) liquefaction necrosis, (3) caseous necrosis, (4) gangrenous necrosis, (5) fibrinoid necrosis, (6) fat necrosis. Once you can memorize the item list, the next step is to memorize individual characteristic, then differentiate them between each other.

For example, coagulation necrosis is due to sudden cutoff of blood supply, leading to protein denaturation. There is preservation of tissue architecture. In contrast, in liquefactive necrosis, tissue hydrolysis occurs, so it becomes soft and liquefied. Caseous necrosis is cause by TB. The resulting necrosis is a combination of coagulation and liquefactive necrosis. Tissue architecture is not entirely preserved, but no liquefaction occurs. Gangrenous necrosis is also cut off of blood supply to extremities or bowel. It can lead to two states, (1) wet gangrene, which like liquefactive necrosis is due to hydrolysis or (2) dry gangrene, which is more like coagulation necrosis. Fibrinoid necrosis occurs on vascular walls and is due to deposition of fibrin-like material due to immune mediated vasculitis. Fat necrosis is due to enzymatic digestion of pancreatic parenchyma or trauma to fat cells.

Memorizing Processes

Memorizing processes involves understanding the different steps in the process first before going through the details. In some cases, you can even group steps that have similar function in the process making it easier to memorize. Only after you have memorized the steps do you begin to study the details of each step. After reviewing the details of each step, you should ask yourself how any modification in the step can lead to pathology.

For example, the coagulation cascade and all the pathology of the coagulation cascade can be studied this way. We know that the coagulation cascade is a series of enzymatic reactions that lead to the production of clotting factors that cascade and end with the production of fibrin from fibrinogen.

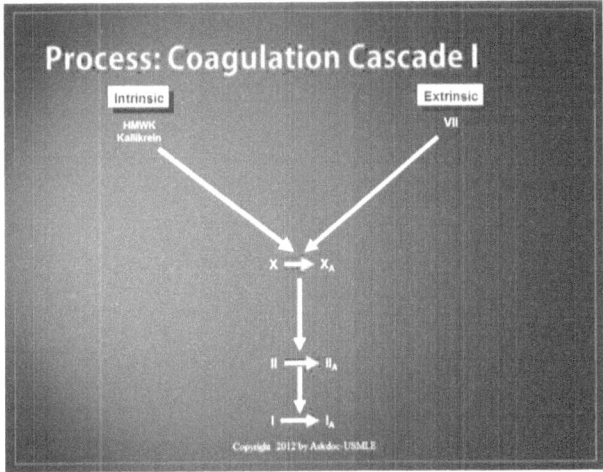

First, we take note of all the steps in the process. Since this is a biochemical process, we start with the key steps then fill in the intermediate steps. A good way of visualizing the coagulation cascade is as a Y with Factor X on the middle. One arm is the intrinsic pathway, the other arm is the extrinsic pathway and the single leg is the final common pathway. The extrinsic pathway starts with Factor VII while the intrinsic pathway starts with Factor XII, HMWK and Kallikrien. The final common pathway goes from factor X to Factor II to Factor I.

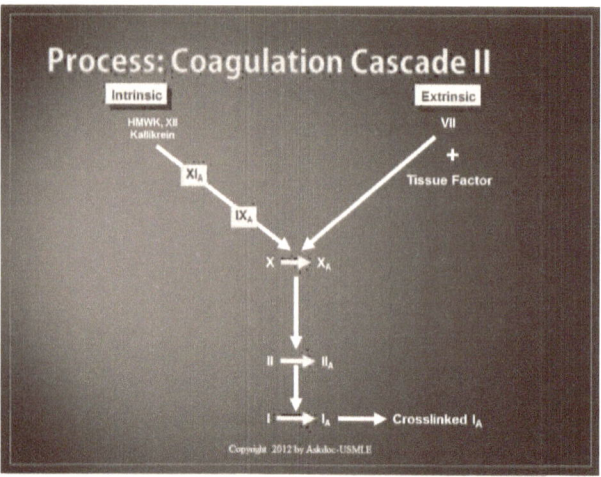

The intermediate step for the intrinsic pathway includes production of factor XI and factor IX. On the extrinsic arm factor VII combines with Tissue factor to produce factor VII A. Meanwhile at the end of the final common pathway, fibrin is cross-linked.

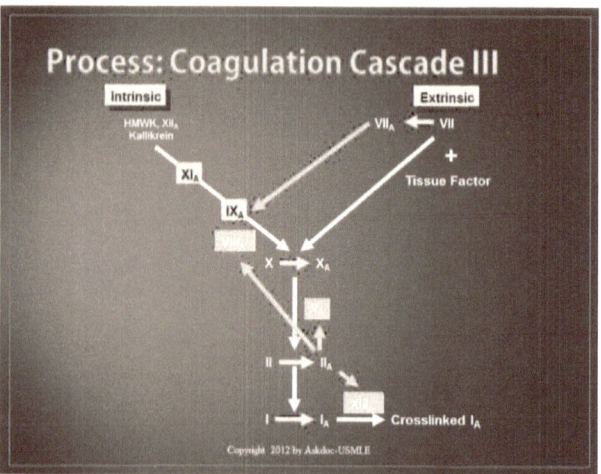

Once we have outlined the different steps of the process, we put in the steps that either speed up or slows down or reverses the process. For example, factor VIIA activates the conversion of factor IX to IX A. Factor VIIIA also activates the conversion of factor IX to IX A. Factor VA activates factor X to XA conversion and factor XIII activates crosslinking of fibrin or factor IA. Without these factors accelerating the process, coagulation will occur thousands of time slower than it does. Factor VIIIA, VA and XIIIA meanwhile is activated by factor IIA or Thrombin.

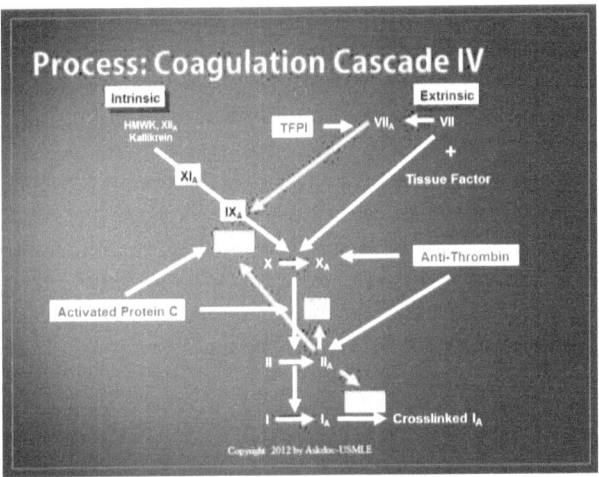

Last step is to fill in the factors that slow down or reverses the process. TFPI or Tissue Factor Plasma Inhibitor slows down VIIA production. Activated Protein C acts on factor VIIIA and Factor VA slowing down the cascade. Anti-thrombin slows down factor X and Thrombin production.

Now that you have memorized the steps in the cascade, the next step is to study the details of each step. For example where each factor is produced. Which factor is vitamin K dependent, etc. It also pays to understand what pathology can happen if any of the factor gets modified, either stop functioning or accelerates its function.

Lastly, fit in the pathology to the proper steps in the process. Then study the details of each pathology. For example, Classic hemophilia is due to factor VIII deficiency. Factor VIII is important in the extrinsic pathway. Another example is Vitamin K deficiency. It results in deficiency of factor II, VII, IX, X. Meanwhile Factor V Leiden is due to a defective factor V which cannot be deactivated by activated protein C. This leads to thrombophilia or hypercoagulability.

Reviewing Concepts from Different Context

I have often been asked the question, if I studied a concept before in a different part of the book, and I encounter the same concept in another part of the book, should I skip it or not. The answer is you should study every concept in the context you found it. If the same concept is found in 5 different contexts, then study it in those contexts. Otherwise during the exam, when the concept comes out in a context you did not study it from, at best you waste time analyzing and trying to recall the concept in the context you studied and reorienting it to the context of the question. At worse, you fail to reorient to the new context of the question, so you fail to answer it.

Integrating Between General Pathology and Systems Pathology

Most of the integration you will be doing within pathology is between general pathology and systems pathology. General pathology discusses pathologic process that are true for all systems in general or compares pathologic process that occur cross different organ systems and tissues. Systems pathology on the other hand covers pathologic processes that are specific to individual systems and tissues. Integrating general pathology and systems pathology means not only knowing general pathologic processes, but understanding how these processes find expression in individual organs and tissues. For example, tissue necrosis happens to all organs and tissues and yet the specific pathologic process in individual organ differs. Coagulation necrosis in the heart vs. liquefaction necrosis in the brain. Even the etiologic factors causing necrosis can cause different pathology. Gangrenous necrosis of bacterial infection vs. caseous necrosis of TB infection vs. fat necrosis due to action of digestive enzymes.

Answering Chapter by Chapter Quiz using Robbin's Review of Pathology

During the first revision, it is important to insure that you are studying pathology the right way. And if there is a problem, you need to correct it as early in your review as possible. So you need to take a quiz at the end of each chapter to insure that you have understood, retained and be able to recall enough of that chapter before moving to the next. Remember the main gauge of your progress is not how much you have read, but how much you have retained and can recall.

For Pathology, we use the quiz at the end of each chapter of Robbin's Review of Pathology and my online q bank for that purpose. Try to score at least 80%, otherwise reread the chapter before attempting to retake the quiz. If you get at least 80% move on to the next chapter.

If you are enrolled in my online Pathology course, the correct sequence is to do the online quiz first. If you score at least 80%, proceed to Robbins Review of Pathology. If not then revise the chapter again. Then retake the online quiz before taking Robbins. You also need to score at least 80% in Robbins, otherwise, you review the whole chapter one more time and retake Robbins.

Your revision for Pathology is more intense than for other subjects. The prime reason is the importance of the subject for the USMLE Step 1. Therefore, it pays to spend more time mastering Pathology.

Studying Clinical Vignettes

With the increasing clinical slant of the USMLE Step 1, more and more questions are appearing in clinical vignette format. Questions in clinical vignette format require you to be able to diagnose a case first before answering basic science question about the case. In order to be able to diagnose clinical vignettes, you need to know the signs and symptoms of the disease as well as pertinent laboratory tests.

In Step 1, only pathology contains information about the signs and symptoms of most of the diseases in detail. Other subjects may occasionally mention them, but only very seldom. With the exception of Microbiology, except that Microbiology covers only infectious disease and nothing else. Therefore you need to study signs and symptoms during your review of pathology.

Reading up from Robbin's Pathologic Basis of Diseases on Topics You Find Hard to Understand

Unless you did a formal learning phase, there might be some topics that you did not understand very well during your first revision. In that case, you need to read up the topics in a basic text. For Pathology, nothing beats Robbin's Pathologic Basis for Diseases in terms of detailed explanation. Therefore, it is highly recommended that you use this text for this purpose. ■

CHAPTER 30

SECOND REVISION OF PATHOLOGY

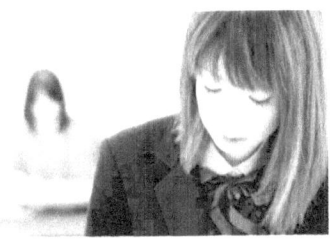

Continue to Memorize All Topics Covered in First Revision

The main purpose of the second revision is to try to integrate related topics between different subjects together. For pathology, this includes anatomy, physiology, biochemistry and pharmacology.

For the second revision, you should continue memorizing what you have studied in the first revision. The purpose is to cement what you have memorized in the first revision. Don't just read through them; try to recite them out loud without looking at them.

Integrate Anatomy, Physiology and Biochemistry into Pathology

The best way to do your integration is to first integrate structure and function by integrating anatomy and physiology. Then integrate relevant topics in biochemistry into anatomy and physiology. Then integrate all three into pathology and the last step is to integrate pathology to pharmacology taking note of specific physiologic and biochemical processes affected by the drugs that may cause further pathology.

A good example is arachidonic acid metabolism leading to two pathways, (1) cyclo-oxygenase pathway and (2) lipo-oxygenase pathway. The cyclo-oxygenase pathway leads to production of the Prostaglandins while the lipo-oxygenase pathway leads to the production of leukotrienes. Two important prostaglandins produced include prostacyclin and thromboxane A2 which are very important components in clotting. Meanwhile, the leukotrienes are important in producing chronic asthma.

The relative balance between prostacyclin and thromboxane A2 is important in the pathogenesis of blood clots that can cause myocardial infarction or cerebrovascular occlusions. Prostacyclin is produced mainly by the endothelial cells lining blood vessel and has anti-thrombotic properties. Meanwhile, thromboxane A2 is produced by platelets and is pro-thrombotic. Damage to endothelial cell can decrease production of prostacyclin while at the same the exposed materials from the damaged endothelial cells can activate platelets, causing release of thromboxane A2 leading to clotting which can result in an MI or CVA.

This is the basis for the use of aspirin in the prevention of MI and in post-stroke patients. Aspirin acts by irreversibly inactivating cyclo-oxygenase. This causes the production of both prostacyclin and thromboxane A2 to stop. However, since prostacyclin is produced in endothelial cells which have an active nucleus, it will start producing cyclo-oxygenase again in a matter of hours and therefore prostacyclin. On the other hand platelets have no active nuclear material, therefore once cyclo-oxygenase is inactivated; there is no way for platelets to produce thromboxane A2 until megakaryocytes in the bone marrow are released into circulation as platelets.

The most important factor for this phenomenon is the fact that aspirin binds irreversibly to cyclo-oxygenase, therefore deactivating it permanently. On the other hand, most NSAIDs binds with cyclo-oxygenase reversibly and therefore will not deactivate it permanently. Once the effect wears off, both prostaglandins are produced. Hence, NSAIDs are not use for this purpose. This is also the main reason why aspirin is given in small doses. Large doses mean longer duration of action. Which means that the new cyclo-oxygenase produced by the endothelial cells will continue to be deactivated, thus negating the differential in response between endothelial cells and platelets to the effect of aspirin.

The phenomenon of aspirin-induced asthma can also be explained by the arachidonic acid metabolism. (This is an example of a pathology caused by a drug used for treating another condition.) A patient suffering from chronic pain due to rheumatoid arthritis is given aspirin or NSAIDs. This blocks the cyclo-oxygenase pathway. However, the chronic inflammation causing the pain continues to stimulate the arachidonic acid metabolism pathway. The excess arachidonic acid produced is now forced to go through the lipo-oxygenase pathway, thus increasing leukotriene production and triggering asthma or other anaphylactic reactions. You can give drugs that deactivate the lipo-oxygenase pathway, but that is not the best solution. As more arachidonic acid builds up, the increased concentration will force the reaction in favor of the cyclo-oxygenase pathway, leading to less effective pain relief. The best treatment will be to shut down production of arachidonic acid altogether by using steroids.

The basis for recommending the use of omega-3 fatty acid in order to reduce chances of MI can also be explained by the arachidonic acid metabolism pathway. Arachidonic acid is produced from fatty acids found in lipids that make up the cell membrane. In this case phosphatidylinositol. The fatty acid carbon backbone in humans are normally omega-6. It refers to the double bond on the carbon backbone. Human enzymes can only put the double bond on the 6th carbon. Algaes however, are able to put double bonds on the 3rd carbon and these fatty acids are called omega 3 fatty acids. Fish eat Algaes and therefore, these types of fatty acids are found in fishes, especially oily fish like salmons. The reason omega 3 fatty acids are better than omega 6 fatty acids is that the endpoint of arachidonic acid metabolism through the cyclo-oxygenase pathway for omega 3 is thromboxane A3 and not thromboxane A2. Thromboxane A3 has lower pro thrombotic activity compared to the A2 variety.

Integrate Pathology into Pharmacology

All pathology is due to the disruption of an anatomic structure or a physiologic or biochemical process. The role of pharmacology is to restore function or compensate for any loss of function due to pathologic processes. These drugs by themselves may lead to additional pathology. Integrating pathology into pharmacology involves understanding how these drugs affect or modify the pathologic process and whether they can cause additional pathology.

Use Pathology Flashcards

At this point you can start using pathology flashcards to increase your ability to recall the concepts better and faster. You can use Askdoc's High Yield Flashcard Review for Pathology or make your own using the topics in my notes or BRS Pathology.

I do not recommend you use BRS Pathology Flashcards unless you rewrite them. The best type of flashcards to improve retention and recall are flashcards that contain one point per card. So a topic with multiple points need to be placed in separate cards.

Use Only Study Notes and Outline Notes

If you are using my notes, then use the notes only. By this time you should not be referring to textbooks if you did your first revision correctly. You should have corrected any deficiency of the learning phase and covered any topics you did not understand in the first revision.

Make use of the outline notes primarily, trying to remember the details and only glancing at the study notes if you can't recall all the details. This will help cement your retention of the materials.

If you are using BRS Pathology or other books. Then try to read the headings and subheadings in bold print and try to recall the details. Glance at the details only if you can't remember them.

Use Per Subject Quiz like Kaplan Q Book

For the second revision, test your mastery of pathology by using per subject quiz like Kaplan Q book. Aim for at least 80% or higher. ■

CHAPTER 31

THIRD REVISION OF PATHOLOGY

Continue Memorizing all Topics Covered in First Revision

For the third revision, the main purpose is to cover your weak points. At this stage you are doing online Q Banks already as part of your Test Preparation Phase. You use it also to spot weak points and cover them.

You need to continue to memorize all the topics you covered in the first revision. Again, don't just read through them, try to recite them out loud without reading your notes. This will improve your retention and recall of the topics.

Continue Memorizing Integrated Topics You Wrote in Your Notes

It is also very important to continue memorizing the integrated topics you covered in your second revision. You should have written these integrated topics in the margins of your notes so you can refer to them without having to read through everything all over again.

Use Outline Notes Primarily and Try to Recall Details in Study Notes without Reading It

Just like on your second revision, use the outline notes primarily, trying to recall what is in the study notes without looking at them. This will improve your retention of what you have studied. If you are using BRS Pathology or other reviewers, then look at the headings and subheadings only and try to recall the details without reading them.

Continue Using Pathology Flashcards

You should continue to improve your retention of what you have studied and improve your ability to recall them randomly. Continue using flashcards for this purpose.

Use Online Q Banks to Determine What Weak Points need to be Covered

At this point in your revision, you should be doing online qbanks as part of your test preparation phase. Use the results of the q bank to pinpoint your weak areas. Study your weak areas one more time. You still cover everything you studied before at least once. But try to go through your weak points one extra round.

Watch out for integrated topic that you failed to cover in your second revision. Usually a lot of questions in the q bank cover integrated topics. If you discover any new integrated topic in the q bank that you have not studied before, don't just study the answers to the question, go back and cover the integrated topic through your notes. The reason is most integrated topic has multiple points that need to be integrated. An integrated topic question in the qbank may cover only one point of let's say 10 points of that topic. If you just study the question, you know only 1 point and not 10. If an actual question on that topic comes out in the actual exam, it may be based on a different point of the same concept, which you did not cover.

■

CHAPTER 32

HIGH YIELD REVIEW OF PATHOLOGY

High Yield Review is very different from the standard prep you just went through. In high yield review, you concentrate on covering only the highest yield material that will come out in the exam. At this stage you have finished your standard prep which means you have basically covered both high yield and low yield material in Physiology. What we want to do now is make sure that what you remember best is the highest yield information.

For this high yield review, your choice of study material include my outline notes on Pathology, First Aid for the USMLE Step 1 - Section on Pathology or Askdoc's High Yield Flashcard Review for Pathology. You should be doing this within the last two weeks before you sit for the examination.

The best combination is to read through my outline notes in pathology. Then go through the flashcards for a quick recall exercise. ■

***

unit 5

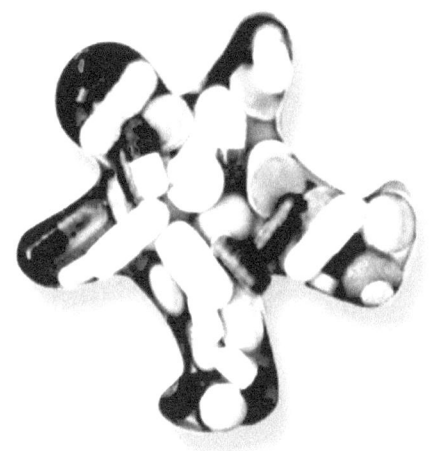

How to Review Pharmacology

CHAPTER 33
INTRODUCTION

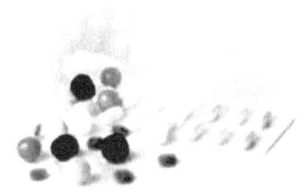

Pharmacology is An Important Subject

Pharmacology is one of the big three and therefore a very important subject. Failure to do well in Pharmacology can be troublesome. It is important that you study pharmacology in the right level of detail. Many times, some of my students decided that they will only study pharmacology superficially using First Aid or Kaplan's Medical Essentials and wonder they can't pass Step 1.

Pharmacology Involves Memorizing a Lot Of Drugs

The main difficulty of reviewing pharmacology is the sheer number of drugs you have to memorize and the amount of detail you need to know about each drug. However, there is a method where you can memorize a little over a hundred drugs and yet be able to answer questions on hundreds of them. We will discuss how you can do that later.

You also need to integrate all these drugs to physiology, biochemistry and pathology. A lot of integrated questions on these topics are included in the exam. ■

CHAPTER 34

STUDY MATERIALS IN PHARMACOLOGY

Study materials for pharmacology can be divided into texts, reviewers, flashcards and q banks.

Textbooks includes Katzung's Basic and Clinical Pharmacology

Reviewers include

- Askdoc's Pharmacology Notes - Study Notes, Outline Notes, Summary Notes
- Lippincott's Illustrated Review of Pharmacology
- Katzung and Trevor's Pharmacology: Examination and Board Review
- Kaplan's Lecture Notes - Section on Pharmacology
- NMS Pharmacology
- First Aid - Section on Pharmacology

Flashcards include

- Askdoc's High Yield Flashcards for Pharmacology
- Pharmcards

Q banks include

- Kaplan's Q Book - Section on Pharmacology
- Kaplan's Online Q Bank - Section on Pharmacology
- USMLE World Online Q Bank - Section on Pharmacology

We will discuss the more important study materials in more detail.

Askdoc's Notes on Pharmacology - Study Notes, Outline Notes, Summary Notes

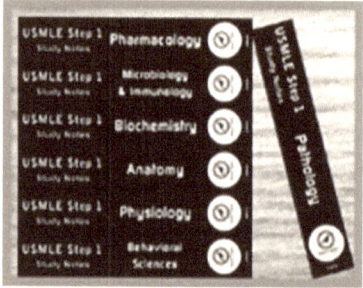

Askdoc's Notes on Pharmacology are the recommended study material for the course. The notes follow all the study methodologies and principles of learning taught in the course. The Study Notes cover all the topics that will be tested in the exam. It covers both low yield and high yield topics. The Outline Notes cover the high yield topics for high yield review. The Summary Notes contain instructions and explanations on how to study each chapter properly.

Lippincott's Illustrated Review of Pharmacology

This is a very good book to understand Pharmacology. Its discussion goes to the basics of Pharmacology. It can be used as a short textbook for Pharmacology, but is also needed for the Mastery Phase as it has detailed discussions on Prototype drugs and some of the major variants of the drugs. The biggest weak point of this book is that it does not cover all the drugs that will come out in the exam. However, using this along with little Katzung will cover all you need to do well in Pharmacology. Another main point is that paired with Lippincott's Illustrated Review of Biochemistry, it covers some integrated topics helpful in the exam.

Katzung and Trevor's Pharmacology:

Examination and Board Review

Also called little Katzung. Hands down one of the best books for reviewing Pharmacology. It has a list of drugs after each chapter. The prototypes you need to master, the major derivatives you have to know and other drugs that you just need to know are part of the same subclass as the prototype. There are great review questions at the end of each chapter which can be the basis for your own per chapter quiz for the first revision. Only problem is that it's discussion of the prototype drugs is not as detailed as it should be. Therefore pairing it with Lippincott's Illustrated Review of Pharmacology is ideal.

Katzung's Basic and Clinical Pharmacology

Also called Big Katzung. Nice big book that covers all the materials superbly. Pharmacology equivalent of Big Robbin's. Personally, I had used little Katzung and Lippincott primarily, but occasionally find myself going to Big Katzung. As with Big Robbin's this book can help you score high in Pharmacology. But again time constraint and the size of the book may make it difficult to use this book for primary review. As with Big Robbin's better to use it as occasional reference for really tough to understand topics.

NMS Pharmacology

Has all the disadvantages of Lippincott's without any of its good points. It covers a lot of drugs in detail, a lot of times with too much detail and yet is missing a lot of essential drugs that will come out of the exam. Don't bother to think about even using it.

Kaplan's Lecture Notes - Section on Pharmacology

Great coverage of Pharmacology but far, far inferior to little Katzung. Like little Katzung, you would need to supplement with Lippincott and refer to Big Katzung for more difficult topic. Next best review book to Little Katzung, but why bother when you have Little Katzung. I went through it about a week before the exam just to find if I missed out on anything important. Found out I didn't.

First Aid - Section on Pharmacology

As with everything about First Aid, it's a good high yield review for the last two weeks of the exam. Although it covers most of the drugs that will come out in the exam, it lacks enough details for a thorough review of Pharmacology. Never use alone.

PharmCards

Flashcards are an excellent way to help you recall lots of unrelated information, especially list of drugs. Given the fact that you need to practice random recall in an exam like the USMLE, it is even more important that you use flashcards to help you with that. However, the best flashcards should have only one point per card. So a topic with several important points need to be in several flashcards not one. Most commercial flashcards including PharmCards contain too many topics per card. Better to build your own or use my High Yield Flashcard for Pharmacology in my site. ■

CHAPTER 35

WHAT TO STUDY IN PHARMACOLOGY

Pharmacology is one of the big three in Step 1, therefore a very important subject. However, it's also a very big subject with potentially thousands of different drugs. Fortunately, you don't have to study all the drugs and there are ways for you to cover all the important drugs without memorizing all the details of all the drugs. We will discuss that when we discuss in detail how to study pharmacology.

Here we will try to discuss how to determine what is important in pharmacology. Again you don't have to study all the drugs nor all the details about the drugs. We need to understand that USMLE wants you to know how drugs work in treating patients. They also want us to understand that drugs are not completely safe, so we have to be aware that using drugs for treatment can have potential to harm the patients. And drug combinations can potentiate their effects whether for good or ill.

The following are guidelines on where to concentrate your studies. Basic pharmacology like pharmacokinetics and pharmacodynamics are of medium importance. There will be a few questions on them with 2 to 3 questions requiring some calculation. For pharmacotherapeutics, the drugs are divided into classes and subclasses under each class. Although all classes of drugs will be covered in the exam. The highest yield classes include the drugs affecting the nervous system, the cardiovascular system, the endocrine system and chemotherapeutic drugs. All other classes are of medium importance.

These classes, for example diuretics are divided further into subclasses, like thiazides, loop diuretics, osmotic diuretics, etc. you of course need to know the basic effect of each class of drugs. For each subclass, you need to know and master very well the prototype drugs. You also need to know the major variants. There are minor variants and for that you only need to know they belong to the same subclass as the prototype.

Now for each drug the most important thing you need to know are the following:

- **Mechanism of action**
- **Adverse effect and Toxicities**
- **Major Drug interactions**
- **Mechanisms of Drug Resistance**
- **Main Use**

You still need to know other feature of the drugs including other uses, metabolism, and route of administration. But they are of medium importance. Dosage is not very important in Step

As we said before, we cannot list all the drugs that you need to study or the level of detail you need to study for each drug. You can however use reviewers which covers the drugs that the author thinks will come out in the exam at the right level of detail for each drug. My pharmacology notes cover what I think will come out in the exam. ■

CHAPTER 36

FIRST REVISION OF PHARMACOLOGY

How to Review Pharmacology

Pharmacology is composed of both list of concepts you need to memorize and processes you need to understand and memorize. The drugs are usually divided into classes. These drug classes are divided into subclasses. Drug classes are grouped together according to the system they affect most although a lot of drugs affect multiple systems.

The lists of drugs we need to study are tremendous. You need to memorize the subclasses under each class. Then the prototype drug under each subclass, then its major derivatives and minor drugs under each subclass. You need to memorize the list of characteristics of each drug. Then processes that include mechanism of action, how adverse reaction happens, etc.

The main review material we will use is Askdoc's Notes on Pharmacology. Alternative is to combine Lippincott's Illustrated Review of Pharmacology with Katzung and Trevor's Pharmacology: Examination and Board Review.

Memorize Headings and Subheadings

First, you need to organize the different classes and subclasses of drugs in your head by memorizing the headings and subheadings. For each class of drugs, you need to be able to enumerate the different subclasses, then the prototype drugs under each subclass and the major and minor variants that belong to each subclass.

Understand that each class of drugs act on a specific organ or system and the subclass usually acts on a specific physiologic or biochemical process or is used for a specific pathology. Therefore, by memorizing the drugs that belong to each subclass and class, it is easier to remember in general what each drugs does. Memorizing each individual drug one at a time is not only tedious but confusing.

All discussions of each class or subclass begins with a short discussion of the physiologic or biochemical process the subclass of drugs affect or the pathologic process the drug is used for. This helps you relate the drugs to each other and differentiate where they act and their therapeutic and adverse effect. At this stage, it is sufficient for you to read these short discussions, but when you reach the second revision, you need to read up this processes in physiology, biochemistry and pathology. This not only deepens your understanding for how the processes relate to the drugs, but also help you remember than better and see the big picture. Remember, a drug may affect only a specific step in a process, but modification of that step in the process can affect other steps in the process as well as other processes. A lot of times, the only way to see the whole picture is to review the whole process in detail at the source, whether in physiology biochemistry or pathology.

Integrating and Comparing Drugs from Different Subclasses

So now you have memorized the drugs according to what class and subclass they belong. You have done a short review of the physiologic, biochemical or pathologic process in which the subclass acts on. What next?

The best way to proceed is to first study the prototype drug of each subclass. Study them as detailed as possible. Then try to compare the prototype drugs of each subclass to understand how they differ from each other. A lot of times you will encounter questions that will test whether you know which drugs are best for a specific situation and why. Each subclass of drug are treatment of choice for specific conditions and you need to know what they are.

The next step is to review again the prototype drug for each subclass. Then for each major variant drug in the subclass understand and memorize how they are different from the prototype. The differences usually revolves around their duration of action, route of administration or elimination, side effects, toxicity, etc. this can make them more useful for certain clinical situation than the prototype drugs. Again expect a lot of questions that tests whether you know what differentiates a major variant drug from the prototype and when you need to use them.

Now for the minor variant, there are only two things you need to know. First what subclass they belong to and second, what is the one major difference between that variant and the prototype.

By studying this way, you need to study in detail less than a hundred drugs, but know how to answer questions on hundreds of different drugs.

One of the things you need to be aware of is that sometimes a question is asking if you can differentiate between two subclasses of drugs. However, the answer on the choices may not contain the prototype of that subclass or even its major variant. In cases like that, then the correct answer is the minor variant even though the prototype drug should have been the best answer. But if the choices contain multiple drugs of the same subclass, then the question wants to know if you understand the specific characteristic of each drug. So you need to answer accordingly.

Memorizing List of Concepts

Lists of concepts you need to memorize include the

different subclasses of drugs and the different drugs under each subclass. Basically you need to memorize all the drugs under a subclass first before you even start studying the details of each drug. Once you study the details try to determine the difference between drugs of each sub classes.

Memorizing Processes

Mechanism of action of a drug are mostly process and there are multiple steps in this process. First understand the process as a whole by memorizing all the steps. Once you know the steps in order, only then should you memorize the details of each step. Understand what each step does for the process and what happens if changes are done in any of these steps.

Reviewing Concepts from Different Contexts

There is a need to review concepts in the different context in which they are presented to us. The reason is that the USMLE can ask the questions based on any context. If you study the concept in only one context and then the question presents the concept in a different context, you need to analyse and think through the concept to understand it from the other context before you can answer the question. That takes more time and you need every second you have for the USMLE.

Second is that by reviewing concepts from different context, you not only study the concept again, you increase the total number of relationships between concepts. You are increasing your retention of those concepts by using the principle of relation and repetition.

For example, beta blockers are initially discussed under autonomic drugs, where it's various uses are enumerated including how they mediate their action. But when you reach the section on cardiovascular drugs, it's again mentioned in relation to its use in angina and hypertension. It is no problem if questions always appear one way, which is it presents from the point of view of autonomic drugs, then where this autonomic drug is effective. But a lot of times, it can start from the condition being treated like angina and you need to be able to know all the drugs that can treat angina including beta blockers. Knowing it both ways make it easier and faster to think through the answer.

The same holds true between subjects like pharmacology and microbiology when it comes to chemotherapeutic drugs. You can study it from the context of the drug and what organisms it can affect or from the context of the organism and what drugs will affect it. Also whereas discussions in pharmacology about the drug will concentrate more on the characteristics of the drug, discussions in microbiology will center more on how the drug affects the organism.

Answering Chapter by Chapter Quiz in Katzung and Trevor Pharmacology

During the first revision, it is important to insure that you are studying pharmacology the right way. And if there is a problem, you need to correct it as early in your review as possible. So you need to take a quiz at the end of each chapter to insure that you have understood, retained and be able to recall enough of that chapter before moving to the next. Remember the main gauge of your progress is not how much you have read, but how much you have retained and can recall.

For Pharmacology, we use the quiz at the end of each chapter of Katzung for that purpose. Try to score at least 80%, otherwise reread the chapter before attempting to retake the quiz. If you get at least 80% move on to the next chapter.

Reading up in Lippincott's Illustrated Review of Pharmacology on Topics You Find Hard to Understand

Unless you did a formal learning phase, there might be

some topics that you did not understand very well during your first revision. In that case, you need to read up the topics in a basic text. Although Lippincott's Illustrated Review can be considered a reviewer, it has basic discussions in the entire major topic and is fairly easy to understand. ■

CHAPTER 37

SECOND REVISION OF PHARMACOLOGY

Continue to Memorize All Topics Covered in First Revision

The main purpose of the second revision is to try to integrate related topics between different subjects together. For pharmacology, this includes physiology, biochemistry and pathology.

For the second revision, you should continue memorizing what you have studied in the first revision. The purpose is to cement what you have memorized in the first revision. Don't just read through them; try to recite them out loud without looking at them.

Integrating Physiology and Biochemistry into Pharmacology

A lot of drugs primarily affect a step either in a physiologic or biochemical process. It is important to know the details of these physiologic or biochemical process. In Pharmacology, you start with the specific drug and what step in the process it affects. However it also pays to know a specific process in detail and all the drugs that affect the different steps. Again the reason is a question can go either way. Integrating your knowledge both ways will help you answer these types of questions much faster and better.

A good example is diuretics and the nephron. Study the different processes that occur in the nephron. Then which type of diuretics affect what steps in the nephron or specific processes within each step. Only then do you study in detail each of the diuretics discussed.

Integrating Pathology into Pharmacology

Once we understand that pathology is due to the disruption of physiologic or biochemical process leading to dysfunction or even complete loss of function, we need to realize that the body will try to compensate for this dysfunction or loss of function or try to restore it. Pharmacologic intervention aims to do these by acting on specific steps in the physiologic or biochemical process to either compensate for or restore loss of function. Integrating pathology into pharmacology involves understanding at what areas of the pathologic process these drugs are effective and whether they compensate for or restore loss of function. We also need to be aware of course that the drugs themselves can cause significant pathology.

Use Pharmacology Flashcards

At this point you can start using pharmacology flashcards to increase your ability to recall the concepts better and faster. You can use Askdoc's High Yield Flashcard Review for Pharmacology or make your own using the topics in my notes or the key words for key drugs section at the back of Katzung.

I do not recommend you use Pharmcards unless you rewrite them. The best type of flashcards to improve retention and recall are flashcards that contain one point per card. So a topic with multiple points needs to be placed in separate cards.

Use Only Study Notes and Outline Notes

If you are using my notes, then use the notes only. By this time you should not be referring to textbooks if you did your first revision correctly. You should have corrected any deficiency of the learning phase and covered any topics you did not understand in the first revision.

Make use of the outline notes primarily, trying to remember the details and only glancing at the study notes if you can't recall all the details. This will help cement your retention of the materials.

If you are using Katzung or other books. Then try to read the headings and subheadings in bold print and try to recall the details. Glance at the details only if you can't remember them.

Use Per Subject Quiz like Kaplan Q Book

For the second revision, test your mastery of pharmacology by using per subject quiz like Kaplan Q book. Aim for at least 80% or higher. ■

CHAPTER 38

THIRD REVISION OF PHARMACOLOGY

Continue Memorizing all Topics Covered in First Revision

For the third revision, the main purpose is to cover your weak points. At this stage you are doing online Q Banks already as part of your Test Preparation Phase. You use it also to spot weak points and cover them.

You need to continue to memorize all the topics you covered in the first revision. Again, don't just read through them, try to recite them out loud without reading your notes. This will improve your retention and recall of the topics.

Continue Memorizing Integrated Topics you Wrote in Your Notes

It is also very important to continue memorizing the integrated topics you covered in your second revision. You should have written these integrated topics in the margins of your notes so you can refer to them without having to read through everything all over again.

Use Outline Notes Primarily and Try to Recall Details in Study Notes without Reading It

Just like on your second revision, use the outline notes primarily, trying to recall what is in the study notes without looking at them. This will improve your retention of what you have studied. If you are using Katzung or other reviewers, then look at the headings and subheadings only and try to recall the details without reading them.

Using Pharmacology Flashcards

You should continue to improve your retention of what you have studied and improve your ability to recall them randomly. Continue using flashcards for this purpose.

Use Online Q Banks to Determine What Weak Points Need To Be Covered

At this point in your revision, you should be doing online qbanks as part of your test preparation phase. Use the results of the q bank to pinpoint your weak areas. Study your weak areas one more time. You still cover everything you studied before at least once. But try to go through your weak point's one extra round.

Watch out for integrated topic that you failed to cover in your second revision. Usually a lot of questions in the q bank cover integrated topics. If you discover any new integrated topic in the q bank that you have not studied before, don't just study the answers to the question, go back and cover the integrated topic through your notes. The reason is most integrated topic has multiple points that need to be integrated. An integrated topic question in the qbank may cover only one point of let's say 10 points of that topic. If you just study the question, you know only 1 point and not 10. If an actual question on that topic comes out in the actual exam, it may be based on a different point of the same concept, which you did not cover. ■

CHAPTER 39
HIGH YIELD REVIEW OF PHARMACOLOGY

High Yield Review is very different from the standard prep you just went through. In high yield review, you concentrate on covering only the highest yield material that will come out in the exam. At this stage you have finished your standard prep which means you have basically covered both high yield and low yield material in Pharmacology. What we want to do now is make sure that what you remember best are the highest yield information.

For this high yield review, your choice of study material include my outline notes on Pharmacology, First Aid for the USMLE Step 1 - Section on Pharmacology or Askdoc's High Yield Flashcard Review for Pharmacology. You should be doing this the last two weeks before you sit for the examination.

The best combination is to read through my outline notes in pharmacology. Then go through the flashcards for a quick recall exercise. ■

**

unit 6

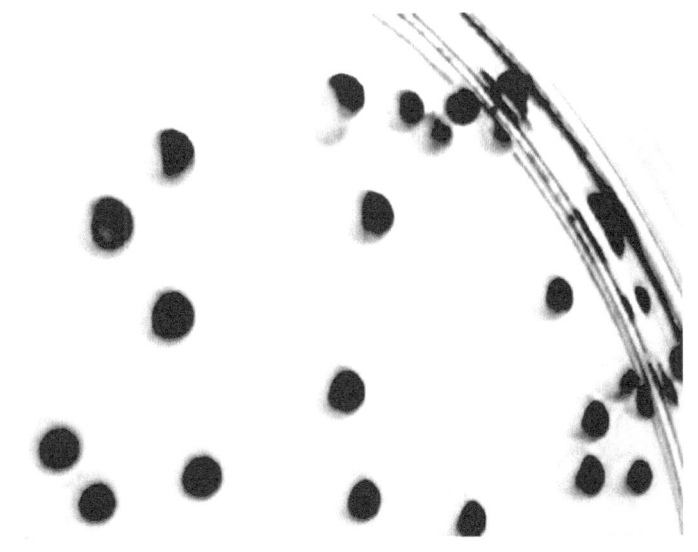

How to Review Microbiology and Immunology

CHAPTER 40
INTRODUCTION

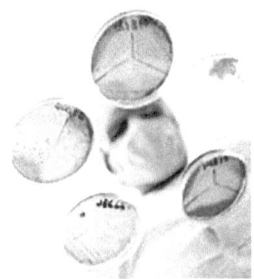

Microbiology and Immunology is An Important Subject

Microbiology and Immunology is one of the big three and therefore a very important subject. Failure to do well in Microbiology can cause trouble later on in your prep. It is important that you study this subject in the right level of detail.

The main difficulty of reviewing microbiology is twofold. First is the sheer number of organisms you have to memorize and the amount of detail you need to know about each them. Second is that immunology is a bit complicated and a lot of people find it hard to understand. ■

CHAPTER 41
STUDY MATERIALS FOR MICROBIOLOGY

Study materials for microbiology and immunology can be divided into texts, reviewers, flashcards and q banks.

Textbooks - none
Reviewers include
- Askdoc's Microbiology and Immunology Notes - Study Notes, Outline Notes, Summary Notes
- Microbiology and Immunology: A Review by Levinson and Jawetz
- Kaplan's Lecture Notes - Section on Microbiology and Immunology
- NMS Microbiology
- First Aid - Section on Microbiology and Immunology

Flashcards include
- Askdoc's High Yield Microbiology and Immunology Flashcards
- Microcards

Q banks include
- Kaplan's Q Book - Section on Microbiology and Immunology
- Kaplan's Online Q Bank - Section on Microbiology and Immunology
- USMLE World Online Q Bank - Section on Microbiology and Immunology

We will discuss the more important study materials in more detail.

Askdoc's Notes on Microbiology and Immunology - Study Notes, Outline Notes and Summary Notes

Askdoc's Notes on Microbiology and Immunology are the recommended study material for the course. The notes follow all the study methodologies and principles of learning taught in the course. The Study Notes cover all the topics that will be tested in the exam. It covers both low yield and high yield topics. The Outline Notes cover the high yield topics for high yield review. The Summary Notes contain instructions and explanations on how to study each chapter properly.

Microbiology and Immunology: A Review by Levinson and Jawetz

This is probably one of the best books you can find for a comprehensive review of Microbiology with great coverage of Immunology to boot. There are questions at the end of the chapters to act as per chapter quizzes for the mastery phase. Although there are no explanations to answers, you can consult relevant chapters for the explanations. When I used this book for my own review, I did not need to refer to any textbooks since the explanations are done quite well. And to think Microbiology was my weakest subject in medical school.

NMS Microbiology

Although in general, far inferior to Levinson and Jawetz, it has superb coverage of chemotherapeutic drugs. It discusses chemotherapeutic drugs from the point of view of Microbiology rather than Pharmacology. Whereas Pharmacology discusses more about characteristics of the drug and mentions general effect of the drug on organisms, discussions here concentrate on the effect of the drugs on organisms in more detail.

Kaplan Lecture Notes - Section on Microbiology and Immunology

Very good coverage of Microbiology and Immunology although still far inferior to Levinson and Jawetz. Can be used as substitute for Levinson and Jawetz if necessary. It has a very good presentation of differential microbiology. Went through it about two weeks before the exam, but didn't really miss anything using Levinson and Jawetz.

First Aid - Section on Microbiology and Immunology

As with everything First Aid, best used as a high yield review last two weeks before, the exam. Covers all the topics that may come out in the exam, but lacks enough detail to serve as a comprehensive review of Microbiology and Immunology. Never use alone.

MicroCards

Flashcards are an excellent way to train recall of micro-organisms. Especially for the USMLE, you need to be able to recall the organisms randomly. However, in order to train recall effectively, each card must contain only one point about a topic. If a topic has several points, it must be organized in separate cards. Most commercial flashcards like MicroCards contain too many topics per card. You are better off constructing your own or using my online High Yield Flashcard Review of Microbiology and Immunology. ∎

CHAPTER 42

WHAT TO STUDY FOR MICROBIOLOGY

Microbiology and Immunology is one of the big three in Step 1. And a very important one. It's also a very big subject with lots of organisms to memorize. Immunology is also very complicated with lots of complex processes going on. Fortunately, we don't really have to study all the bugs nor all the details on the bugs we need to study. There is no way for me to list everything you need to study in Microbiology and Immunology in this book. However, you can use my reviewer on Microbiology and Immunology if you want to know what I think will come out in the examination.

We know that the USMLE wants to know if you understand basic medical sciences applied to clinical practice. Therefore, the materials you need to concentrate on are those that will apply to clinical practice. Microbiology includes a lot of topic that are of primary interest to microbiologist in a laboratory or research setting. These topics are considered of lesser importance as far as the USMLE is concerned.

First, most questions will cover Bacteriology, Virology and Immunology. Very few questions will cover mycology and parasitology. In bacteriology and virology, not all organisms will be covered in detail and some not at all. The more common organisms that cause pathology will be tested in more detail than organisms that rarely cause human disease.

For each of the microorganism, you need to master pathogenesis and host response, treatment of choice, mechanisms of drug action and resistance. You also need to know the clinical signs and symptoms, mode of transmission and how to diagnose or confirm the diagnosis.

Less important are classification of the organisms. Know the general classification, i.e. gram + rods, etc or for the more important viruses, whether they are DNA or RNA and some of the major classes like retrovirus for AIDS, etc. otherwise classification are low yield. Single-stranded, double-stranded, linear, circular, etc. are very low yield.

For Immunology, most important is to understand the immune response of the body. Immune response is complicated process and you need to understand how these process works. Different processes include passive vs. active, innate vs acquired and humoral vs. cell-mediated immunity. You also need to know the diseases of immunity. Overall, immunology is the most high-yield, followed by bacteriology, then virology. ■

CHAPTER 43
FIRST REVISION OF MICROBIOLOGY AND IMMUNOLOGY

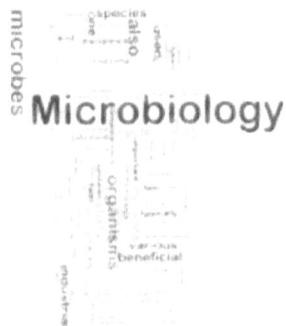

How to Study Microbiology and Immunology

Although microbiology and immunology is treated as one subject, there is a difference in the way they are studied. Microbiology consists of a lot of organisms you need to memorize. Each organism consists of lots of characteristics you need to memorize. They are basically lists of properties of each organism. Processes in microbiology cover the pathophysiology of the diseases and host response.

In contrast, immunology is composed mostly of processes. And since immunology tend to function in an integrated manner; you need to integrate all these processes together to basically understand immunology as a whole.

Another thing, aside from Pathology, Microbiology is the only subject in Step 1 where clinical signs and symptoms are discussed, although it's basically limited to infectious diseases. Therefore, you need to study them for the clinical vignette part of the examination.

Memorize Headings and Subheadings

You need to memorize headings and subheadings in order to provide a framework to organize what you know and are going to learn about microbiology. It will also make it easier to recall information later in the exam. Microbiology is organized according to type of organisms. For example, bacteria vs virus vs fungi, etc. Under bacteria, it's divided in gram (+) cocci, gram (-) cocci, gram (+) rods, then gram (-) rods. Most of these classifications group organism with similar characteristics together. Therefore studying them this way can help you recall the information better.

Memorizing List of Concepts

When memorizing a list of items, first memorize all the items in the list. Then go through details of each item. Compare difference between details of each item and memorize that too.

For example, staphylococcus has three important species. (1) s. aureus, (2) s. epidermidis, (3) s. saprophyticus. After memorizing all three, the next step is to study and memorize the details: pathogenesis, epidemiology, mode of transmission, treatment, laboratory detection, etc. Once you have finished with the details, take the extra step of knowing what is the same or different between the items. They are all gram(+) cocci that are catalase positive. But they differ in the disease caused, mode of transmission, epidemiology, treatment, etc. Make sure you know all of them.

Memorizing Processes

Processes in microbiology and immunology usually revolve

around pathophysiology or immunology. When you study processes, it is important to memorize all the steps in the process first. Then go through details of the process before noting all important regulatory steps.

Reviewing Concepts from Different Context

Reviewing concepts from different context is important because a question in the USMLE can ask questions from any context, not just in the context you have memorized it. For example, antibiotics are discussed both in microbiology and pharmacology but in different context. In microbiology, the emphasis is more on the effect of the drug on the organism while in pharmacology, it describes the characteristics of the drugs in more detail. So study them in both contexts because you won't know how the USMLE will ask the question.

Integrating Basic Bacteriology to Clinical Bacteriology

Basic Bacteriology discusses general characteristics of bacteria including general morphology, life cycle, etc. Clinical Bacteriology covers specific characteristics of individual bacteria. It is important to relate the general characteristics of these bacteria to the specific characteristic of each individual bacterium in order to better understand how they differ from each other.

Integrating Basic Virology to Clinical Virology

Same thing holds true with the viruses. Basic Virology discusses general characteristics of viruses including general morphology, life cycle, etc. Clinical Virology covers specific characteristics of individual viruses. It is important to relate the general characteristics of these viruses to the specific characteristic of each individual virus in order to better understand how they differ from each other.

For example, even though all viruses generally follow the same growth cycle, there are individual differences among viruses. In general, all viruses go through the following growth cycle, (1) attachment and penetration, (2) uncoating of viral genome, (3) early viral mRNA synthesis, (4) early viral protein synthesis, (5) viral genome replication, (6) late viral mRNA synthesis, (7) late viral protein synthesis, (8) progeny virion assembly, (9) progeny virion release.

Individual viruses differ in exactly how they carry out these steps. For example, how the viral genome replicates depends on whether they are single-stranded or double-stranded, linear or circular, DNA or RNA, etc. These are important because the USMLE will test whether you know the difference or not.

Answering Chapter by Chapter Quiz in Levinson and Jawetz

During the first revision, it is important to insure that you are studying microbiology and immunology the right way. And if there is a problem, you need to correct it as early in your review as possible. So you need to take a quiz at the end of each section to insure that you have understood, retained and be able to recall enough of that section before moving to the next. Remember the main gauge of your progress is not how much you have read, but how much you have retained and can recall.

For Microbiology and Immunology, we use the quiz at the end of each section of Levinson for that purpose. Try to score at least 80%, otherwise reread the section before attempting to retake the quiz. If you get at least 80% move on to the next chapter. Unlike the other quizzes, there is no explanation to answer. However, you can look at the relevant chapters in Microbiology and Immunology for the explanations.

Studying Clinical Vignettes

With the increasing clinical slant of the USMLE Step 1,

more and more questions are appearing in clinical vignette format. Questions in clinical vignette format require you to be able to diagnose a case first before answering basic science question about the case. In order to be able to diagnose clinical vignettes, you need to know the signs and symptoms of the disease as well as pertinent laboratory tests.

In Step 1, aside from pathology only microbiology contains information about the signs and symptoms of infectious diseases in detail. Other subjects may occasionally mention them, but only very seldom. Therefore you need to study signs and symptoms during your review of microbiology.

Reading up from Levinson and Jawetz on Topics You Find Hard to Understand

Unless you did a formal learning phase, there might be some topics that you did not understand very well during your first revision. In that case, you need to read up the topics in a basic text. Although Levinson and Jawetz Microbiology and Immunology Review can be considered a reviewer, it covers all the major topics in proper detail and is fairly easy to understand. ∎

CHAPTER 44
SECOND REVISION OF MICROBIOLOGY AND IMMUNOLOGY

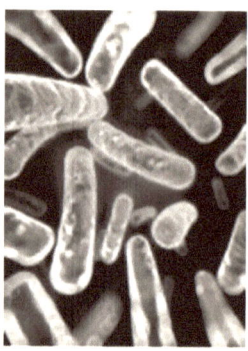

Continue to Memorize All Topics Covered in First Revision

The main purpose of the second revision is to try to integrate related topics between different subjects together. For microbiology and immunology, this includes physiology, biochemistry, pharmacology and pathology.

For the second revision, you should continue memorizing what you have studied in the first revision. The purpose is to cement what you have memorized in the first revision. Don't just read through them; try to recite them out loud without looking at them.

Integrate Physiology and Biochemistry with

Microbiology and Immunology

Most pathology caused by organisms affect physiologic and biochemical process in the body. Metabolism of these organisms is also related to biochemical process. There are short discussion of these processes from within microbiology and immunology, but it pays to read through relevant chapter of physiology and biochemistry to cement your knowledge.

Integrate Microbiology and Immunology with Pathology

Generally, the pathology caused by organisms is discussed within microbiology and immunology itself. However, the discussion in pathology is more detailed. Therefore, you may want to take the extra time to study the infectious disease section of pathology. In my pathology notes, there is no section on infectious disease and therefore you might want to read it up directly from Robbins.

Integrate Microbiology and Immunology with Pharmacology

The main topics you need to integrate between microbiology and pharmacology has to do with chemotherapeutic drugs. Whereas, microbiology tends to discuss in more detail the effect of each drug on the organism, pharmacology will tend to discuss in more detail the characteristics of the drug itself. Plus you need to be able to start with a drug and enumerate all the bugs it is effective against or start with the micro-organism and all the drugs that will affect it.

Use Microbiology and Immunology Flashcards

At this point you can start using microbiology and immunology flashcards to increase your ability to recall the concepts better and faster. You can use Askdoc's High Yield

Flashcard Review for Microbiology or make your own using the topics in my notes or the summary of medically important organism at the back of Levinson and Jawetz..

I do not recommend you use MicroCards unless you rewrite them. The best type of flashcards to improve retention and recall are flashcards that contain only one point per card. So a topic with multiple points needs to be placed in separate cards.

Use Only Study Notes and Outline Notes

If you are using my notes, then use the notes only. By this time you should not be referring to textbooks if you did your first revision correctly. You should have corrected any deficiency of the learning phase and covered any topics you did not understand in the first revision.

Make use of the outline notes primarily, trying to remember the details and only glancing at the study notes if you can't recall all the details. This will help cement your retention of the materials.

If you are using Levinson and Jawetz or other books. Then try to read the headings and subheadings in bold print and try to recall the details. Glance at the details only if you can't remember them.

Use per Subject Quiz like Kaplan Q Book

For the second revision, test your mastery of pharmacology by using per subject quiz like Kaplan Q book. Aim for at least 80% or higher. ■

CHAPTER 45

THIRD REVISION OF MICROBIOLOGY AND IMMUNOLOGY

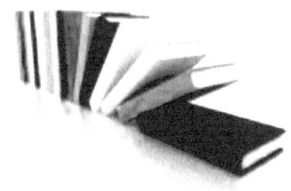

Continue Memorizing All Topics Covered in First Revision

For the third revision, the main purpose is to cover your weak points. At this stage you are doing online Q Banks already as part of your Test Preparation Phase. You use it also to spot weak points and cover them.

You need to continue to memorize all the topics you covered in the first revision. Again, don't just read through them, try to recite them out loud without reading your notes. This will improve your retention and recall of the topics.

Continue Memorizing Integrated Topics You Wrote in Your Notes

It is also very important to continue memorizing the integrated topics you covered in your second revision. You should have written these integrated topics in the margins of your notes so you can refer to them without having to read through everything all over again.

Use Outline Notes Primarily and Try to Recall Details in Study Notes without Reading It

Just like on your second revision, use the outline notes primarily, trying to recall what is in the study notes without looking at them. This will improve your retention of what you have studied. If you are using Kaplan or other reviewers, then look at the headings and subheadings only and try to recall the details without reading them.

Continue Using Microbiology Flashcards

You should continue to improve your retention of what you have studied and improve your ability to recall them randomly. Continue using flashcards for this purpose.

Use Online Q Banks to Determine What Weak Points Need to Be Covered

At this point in your revision, you should be doing online qbanks as part of your test preparation phase. Use the results of the q bank to pinpoint your weak areas. Study your weak areas one more time. You still cover everything you studied before at least once. But try to go through your weak points one extra round.

Watch out for integrated topic that you failed to cover in your second revision. Usually a lot of questions in the q bank cover integrated topics. If you discover any new integrated topic in the q bank that you have not studied before, don't just study the answers to the question, go back and cover the integrated topic through your notes. The reason is most integrated topic has multiple points that need to be integrated. An integrated topic question in the qbank may cover only one point of let's say 10 points of that topic. If you just study the question, you know only 1 point and not 10. If an actual question on that topic comes out in the actual exam, it may be based on a different point of the same concept, which you did not cover. ■

CHAPTER 46

HIGH YIELD REVIEW OF MICROBIOLOGY AND IMMUNOLOGY

High Yield Review is very different from the standard prep you just went through. In high yield review, you concentrate on covering only the highest yield material that will come out in the exam. At this stage you have finished your standard prep which means you have basically covered both high yield and low yield material in Microbiology and Immunology. What we want to do now is make sure that what you remember best is the highest yield information.

For this high yield review, your choice of study material include my outline notes on Microbiology and Immunology, First Aid for the USMLE Step 1 - Section on Microbiology or Askdoc's High Yield Flashcard Review for Microbiology. You should be doing this the last two weeks before you sit for the examination.

The best combination is to read through my outline notes in microbiology. Then go through the flashcards for a quick recall exercise. ■

***

unit 7

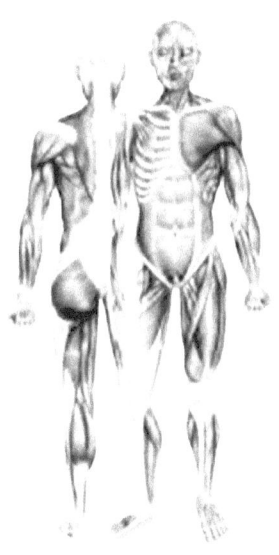

How to Review Anatomy

CHAPTER 47
INTRODUCTION

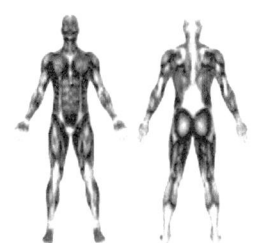

Anatomy is one of the minor subjects and it's probably one of the least studied subjects in Step 1 with the probable exception of Behavioral Science. It consists mostly of list of things you need to memorize. A second problem with anatomy is that although it comprises about 8% of the questions in the exam, the total amount of information you need to study is huge. It's second only to pathology in terms of the number of concepts you need to study and yet pathology comprises as much as 40% of the questions in Step 1.

Anatomy can basically be divided into four sections. (1) Gross Anatomy which is the largest, (2) Neuroanatomy which is also very important, and lastly, (3) Histology and (4) Embryology which is best studied integrated to Gross Anatomy and Neuroanatomy. ■

CHAPTER 48
STUDY MATERIALS IN ANATOMY

Study materials for anatomy can be divided into texts, reviewers, flashcards and q banks.

Textbooks include the following
- Grant's Method of Anatomy
- Gray's Anatomy
- Bloom and Fawcett Histology
- Langman's Embryology
- ***Reviewers include***
- Askdoc's Anatomy Notes - Study Notes, Outline Notes, Summary Notes
- Kaplan's Lecture Notes - Section on Anatomy
- Anatomy Made Ridiculously Simple
- BRS Anatomy
- BRS Neuroanatomy
- High Yield Anatomy
- High Yield Neuroanatomy
- NMS Clinical Anatomy
- First Aid - Section on Anatomy

Flashcards include:
- Askdoc's High Yield Anatomy Flashcards

Q banks include
- Kaplan's Q Book - Section on Anatomy
- Kaplan's Online Q Bank - Section on Anatomy

- USMLE World Online Q Bank - Section on Anatomy

We will discuss the more important study materials in more detail.

Askdoc's Notes on Anatomy - Study Notes, Outline Notes and Summary Notes

Askdoc's Notes on Anatomy are the recommended study material for the course. The notes follow all the study methodologies and principles of learning taught in the course. The Study Notes cover all the topics that will be tested in the exam. It covers both low yield and high yield topics. The Outline Notes cover the high yield topics for high yield review. The Summary Notes contain instructions and explanations on how to study each chapter properly.

Kaplan Lecture Notes on Anatomy

If you just want to pass Anatomy, then this book is adequate. But if you want to really do well, then you need to use another reviewer. Or use this but supplement with the other books. It can be used as main review book for anatomy.

BRS Anatomy

This book covers the main topics that will come out in the exam. Emphasis in clinical anatomy is adequate. There is however a lot of anatomy topics that will not come out in the exam. Can be used as main review book for gross anatomy.

NMS Clinical Anatomy

It covers all the major topics in Anatomy with emphasis on clinical anatomy, which is what is emphasized in Step 1. Main problem is the writing is sometimes obtuse and hard to understand. It also covers a lot of anatomy that will not come out in the examination. Can be used as main review book for for gross anatomy.

High Yield Anatomy

Main advantage of this book is that it covers most of the topics that will one out in the exam and covers very few that will not come out. Main disadvantage is inadequate coverage of the clinical aspect of Anatomy which is important for this exam. Use as supplement.

Grants Method of Anatomy

Good textbook to study regional gross anatomy, but not recommended for reviewing anatomy for Step 1. Too many topics that are not clinically oriented and therefore will not come out in the exam. Suggest using as occasional reference when you need to study a particular topic in more detail.

Gray's Anatomy

Again, a good basic textbook to study gross anatomy but a bad idea to use for reviewing. Use as reference if needed to study a particular topic in more detail.

Anatomy Made Ridiculously Simple

Completely inadequate for understanding and comprehensive review of anatomy. Good mnemonics however and can help you remember stuff. Suggest you use it as a supplement rather than your main reviewer.

Kaplan Lecture Notes on Neuroanatomy

Good enough reviewer although you need a book with more in depth coverage to do well in neuroanatomy. But Kaplan notes are adequate as a main reviewer for Neuroanatomy.

BRS Neuroanatomy

Very good and thorough coverage of neuroanatomy. I personally used this for my own review. Main drawback is that about a third of the topics will not come out in the exam. Best used if aiming for 99 or > 230.

High Yield Neuroanatomy

Good reviewer for Neuroanatomy. Somewhere in between Kaplan notes and BRS Neuroanatomy. Can be used as main reviewer for Neuroanatomy. But if you really want to score high, then better stick to BRS.

Kaplan Lecture Notes on Histology

Barely adequate coverage of histology. If used as main reviewer, try to supplement with pictures.

BRS Histology and Cell Biology

Very good coverage of histology and cell biology. Good discussion on molecular biology topics. However lacks pictures. Most histology questions will contain pictures.

Bloom and Fawcett Histology

Very detailed discussions and lots of pics. Use only as reference. Not recommended as reviewer.

Histology: Text and Atlas

Very good histology pictures. Use as supplement.

Kaplan Lecture Notes on Embryology

Barely adequate coverage of embryology.

Langman's Embryology

Very thorough discussions on embryology. Very good clinical correlation. Very good in depth discussion of molecular biology as related to embryologic development. That said, requires a lot of time commitment. Also discusses a lot of topics that will not come out in the exam. Use only if going for high 99, i.e. > 250. ■

CHAPTER 49

WHAT TO STUDY IN ANATOMY

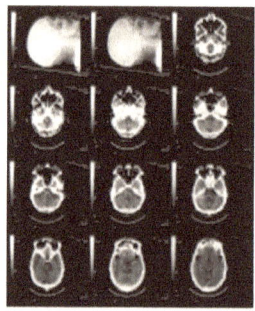

Anatomy is one of the minor subjects. Therefore its importance is not as high as the big three. However, you can't ignore it as it still covers 8 - 10% of the exam. It is surprising that this is considered a minor subject by the USMLE considering the total amount of topics that comprise anatomy is enormous. However, USMLE is more concerned about clinical applications rather than medical facts and anatomy is more about medical facts. There are clinical applications but a large percentage of anatomy has few clinical applications except in some surgical subspecialty. For example, the specific details of insertions and origins of muscles in the hand are very important to a hand surgeon but not very relevant to general practice.

Therefore, expect questions in anatomy not to delve into this level of detail. It is impossible to list everything you need to study in this book. You can use my anatomy notes available thru the course if you want to know what I think will be covered in the exam, or you can use some of the recommended reviewers for this subject. We will discuss here general rules on how to determine what is important for you to study in anatomy.

Anatomy can be divided into four sections. Namely gross anatomy, neuroanatomy, histology and embryology. Most of the questions in anatomy will concentrate on gross anatomy and neuroanatomy with very few questions in histology and embryology.

For gross anatomy, concentrate on anatomy important in pathology. For example, coronary artery circulation is crucial in the pathology of myocardial infarction. Another area to cover are topics important in surgery or orthopedics. For example, anatomy of the inguinal area is important in pathology of hernias. The anatomy of the knee is important in the knee injuries like the unhappy triad of tearing the anterior cruciate ligament, medial meniscus and medial ligament of the knee. Brachial plexus injuries are also high yield. Be able to pinpoint area of injury based on clinical signs and symptoms and vice versa.

For neuroanatomy, concentrate on CNS pathways and syndromes associated with the disruption of these pathways. This includes spinal cord and both cortical and thalamic pathways. Understand that trauma, tumors and disruption of blood supply to these pathways can disrupt these pathways. Cranial nerves and their pathways are also important. For example, cranial nerves to the eye muscles pass through the cavernous sinuses and any pathology of the cavernous sinus can result in palsies of the eye.

CT scans and MRI images of the CNS are also important. However, they are usually classical cases like bleed and tumors. So you don't really have to study the more exotic CT or MRI images.

For histology, cover any histology that is related to pathology. For example, you need to understand the normal histology of cardiac muscle so you can differentiate it from coagulation necrosis of an infarcted myocardial muscle. You also need to cover any histology topic related to molecular biology like laminitis, spectrum, different type of receptors both surface and nuclear, lysosomes, etc.

For embryology, focus should be on embryologic developments that lead to congenital anomalies. For example, cleft lip is the result of failure of fusion of the maxillary and medial nasal processes. ■

CHAPTER 50

FIRST REVISION OF ANATOMY

How to Study Anatomy

Most important thing when studying anatomy is to remember the clinical applications of anatomy. If it's not important clinically, it will not come out in the exam. If you memorize anything in anatomy, know its clinical significance. For example, coronary circulation is important because of myocardial infarction. The brachial plexus is important because of the various orthopedic injuries involving it. The exact origin and insertion of every muscle in the arm and leg may not be as important as their relation to pathology.

Memorize Headings and Subheadings

You need to memorize headings and subheadings in anatomy in order to provide a framework to organize what you know and will learn about anatomy. It will also help you recall what you have studied in a systematic way and increase your chance of scoring better. However, since most questions in anatomy is integrated to pathology, you can opt to organize anatomy under headings in pathology rather than on their own. That is a viable option.

Memorizing List of Concepts

Most of the things you will be studying in anatomy are lists of items you need to memorize. When studying lists of items, it is important to memorize the list first before going through details of each item. Next step is to go through the details, after which you try to take note of the difference between the items in the list.

For example, the lateral cord of the brachial plexus has three nerves. (1) lateral pectoral nerve, (2) musculocutaneous nerve, (3) median nerve. The next step is to memorize the details. Lateral pectoral nerve innervates clavicular head of pectoralis major muscle, musculocutanous nerve, innervates flexor muscles of brachium, etc. And final step differentiate syndrome associated with each nerve injury.

Memorizing Processes

Most of the topics in anatomy are lists of items you need to memorize. Even the few topics that are processes, most of the details are still items you need to memorize. For example respiratory mechanics can be divided into two processes, costal ventilation and diaphragmatic ventilation. Costal ventilation is composed of two types. Normal and forced. Normal costal ventilation involves inspiration and expiration, while forced costal ventilation is also composed of inspiration and expiration, however, the details of each step are different and you need to know the difference.

Integrating Histology and Embryology to Gross Anatomy and Neuroanatomy

It is important that you integrate what you know in histology and embryology to the corresponding topic in gross anatomy and neuroanatomy. Histology is also called microscopic anatomy while embryology is also known as developmental anatomy. You need to be able to relate to the microscopic structure of the organs you are studying as well as how they developed embryologically.

Reading up from NMS Clinical Anatomy on Topics You Find Hard to Understand

How to Master the USMLE Step 1

Unless you did a formal learning phase, there might be some topics that you did not understand very well during your first revision. In that case, you need to read up the topics in a basic text. Although NMS Clinical Anatomy can be considered a reviewer, it has detailed discussions on clinical anatomy and covers them well. ■

CHAPTER 51
SECOND REVISION OF ANATOMY

Continue to Memorize All Topics Covered in First Revision

The main purpose of the second revision is to try to integrate related topics between different subjects together. For anatomy, this includes physiology and pathology.

For the second revision, you should continue memorizing what you have studied in the first revision. The purpose is to cement what you have memorized in the first revision. Don't just read through them; try to recite them out loud without looking at them.

Integrate Anatomy into Physiology

Integrating anatomy into physiology requires structure and function correlation. The best way to do the integration is by system. For example, start with cardiovascular anatomy and histology, correlate with cardiovascular physiology. How does the anatomy of the heart help fulfil its function? How does the specialized heart cells help fulfil its function? How does the anatomy of the heart produce the physiology of heart sounds? These are just examples.

Integrate Anatomy and Physiology into Pathology

After doing structure and function correlation, you can then integrate this with pathology. Continuing the example above, you integrate with cardiovascular pathology. For example, the reason myocardial infarction can be fatal depends on the anatomy of the heart. The coronary circulation, the way the heart muscle is perfused, the anatomy of the bundle of His and the nodes, all contribute to the various pathology of MI. Signs and symptoms of MI is dependent also on both anatomy and physiology. Murmurs occur when specific coronary arteries that supply the valve are hit. Arrhythmia can occur when the coronary artery that supplies the nodes or bundle of His gets affected. How the physiology of the heart is altered due to the pathology caused by MI should also be covered.

Use Anatomy Flashcards

At this point you can start using anatomy flashcards to increase your ability to recall the concepts better and faster. You can use Askdoc's High Yield Flashcard Review for Anatomy or make your own using the topics in my notes.

Use Only Study Notes and Outline Notes

If you are using my notes, then use the notes only. By this time you should not be referring to textbooks if you did your first revision correctly. You should have corrected any deficiency of the learning phase and covered any topics you did not understand in the first revision.

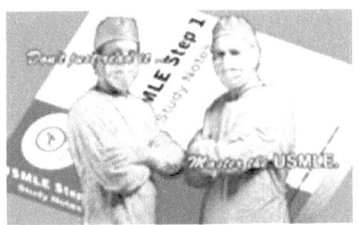

Make use of the outline notes primarily, trying to remember the details and only glancing at the study notes if you can't recall all the details. This will help cement your retention of the materials.

If you are using Kaplan or other books. Then try to read the headings and subheadings in bold print and try to recall the details. Glance at the details only if you can't remember them.

Use Per Subject Quiz like Kaplan Q Book

For the second revision, test your mastery of pharmacology by using per subject quiz like Kaplan Q book. Aim for at least 80% or higher. ■

CHAPTER 52

THIRD REVISION OF ANATOMY

Continue Memorizing All Topics Covered in First Revision

For the third revision, the main purpose is to cover your weak points. At this stage you are doing online Q Banks already as part of your Test Preparation Phase. You use it also to spot weak points and cover them.

You need to continue to memorize all the topics you covered in the first revision. Again, don't just read through them, try to recite them out loud without reading your notes. This will improve your retention and recall of the topics.

Continue Memorizing Integrated Topics You Wrote in Your Notes

It is also very important to continue memorizing the integrated topics you covered in your second revision. You should have written these integrated topics in the margins of your notes so you can refer to them without having to read through everything all over again.

Use Outline Notes Primarily and Try to Recall Details in Study Notes without Reading It

Just like on your second revision, use the outline notes

primarily, trying to recall what is in the study notes without looking at them. This will improve your retention of what you have studied. If you are using Kaplan or other reviewers, then look at the headings and subheadings only and try to recall the details without reading them.

Continue Using Anatomy Flashcards

You should continue to improve your retention of what you have studied and improve your ability to recall them randomly. Continue using flashcards for this purpose.

Use Online Q Banks to Determine What Weak Points need to be Covered

At this point in your revision, you should be doing online qbanks as part of your test preparation phase. Use the results of the q bank to pinpoint your weak areas. Study your weak areas one more time. You still cover everything you studied before at least once. But try to go through your weak points one extra round.

Watch out for integrated topic that you failed to cover in your second revision. Usually a lot of questions in the q bank cover integrated topics. If you discover any new integrated topic in the q bank that you have not studied before, don't just study the answers to the question, go back and cover the integrated topic through your notes. The reason is most integrated topics have multiple points that need to be integrated. An integrated topic question in the qbank may cover only one point of let's say 10 points of that topic. If you just study the question, you know only 1 point and not 10. If an actual question on that topic comes out in the actual exam, it may be based on a different point of the same concept, which you did not cover. ■

CHAPTER 53

HIGH YIELD REVIEW OF ANATOMY

High Yield Review is very different from the standard prep you just went through. In high yield review, you concentrate on covering only the highest yield material that will come out in the exam. At this stage you have finished your standard prep which means you have basically covered both high yield and low yield material in Anatomy. What we want to do now is make sure that what you remember best are the highest yield information.

For this high yield review, your choice of study material include my outline notes on Anatomy, First Aid for the USMLE Step 1 - Section on Anatomy or Askdoc's High Yield Flashcard Review for Anatomy. You should be doing this the last two weeks before you sit for the examination.

The best combination is to read through my outline notes in anatomy. Then go through the flashcards for a quick recall exercise. ■

***

unit 8

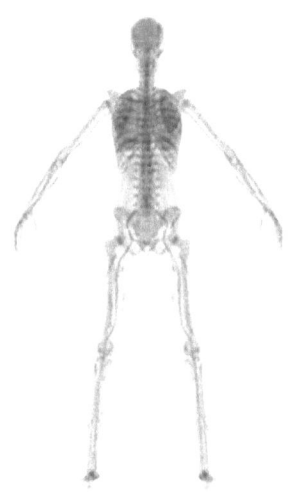

How to Review
Physiology

CHAPTER 54
INTRODUCTION

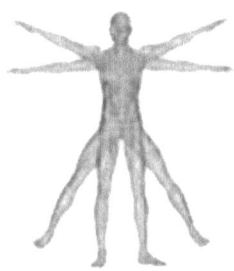

Physiology is considered one of the minor subjects. But its importance is inflated for two reasons. First you need a very good understanding of physiology to do well in Pathology and Pharmacology, two of the most important subjects in Step 1. Second, about a third of pathophysiology is discussed in physiology rather than in pathology. Although pathophysiology is technically filed in pathology, some of the topics are covered in physiology and you need to study them as well as the pathophysiology in pathology.

One of the most important things you have to know about physiology is that most of it involves processes. Although biochemistry also involves a lot of processes, the main difference is that while all the steps in physiologic processes is more or less important, in biochemical processes, only key steps are important. You must emphasize in your study the understanding of how these processes work and that disruption of the steps in the process can result in pathology.

CHAPTER 55

STUDY MATERIALS IN PHYSIOLOGY

Study materials for physiology can be divided into texts, reviewers, flashcards and q banks.

Textbooks include the following
- Guyton's Physiology
- Ganong's Physiology
- Physiology by Linda Costanza

Reviewers include
- Askdoc's Physiology Notes - Study Notes, Outline Notes, Summary Notes
- Kaplan's Lecture Notes - Section on Physiology
- BRS Physiology
- NMS Physiology
- First Aid - Section on Physiology
- **Flashcards** include Askdoc's High Yield Physiology Flashcards

Q banks include
- Kaplan's Q Book - Section on Physiology
- Kaplan's Online Q Bank - Section on Physiology
- USMLE World Online Q Bank - Section on Physiology

We will discuss the more important study materials in more detail.

Askdoc's Notes on Physiology - Study Notes, Outline Notes and Summary Notes

Askdoc's Notes on Physiology are the recommended study material for the course. The notes follow all the study methodologies and principles of learning taught in the course. The Study Notes cover all the topics that will be tested in the exam. It covers both low yield and high yield topics. The Outline Notes cover the high yield topics for high yield review. The Summary Notes contain instructions and explanations on how to study each chapter properly.

BRS Physiology

Very good coverage of physiology. However, if you are poor in physiology, BRS physiology may not be enough. You will need to refer to the texts or NMS for more thorough coverage. Very good as outline notes.

NMS Physiology

An extremely dense book, however good enough to serve as a main textbook if you are poor in physiology. However, there are parts that are very hard to read and understand. It has a very solid coverage of Acid-Base physiology, but weak in cardiology and neurology. Lots of discussions on pathophysiology which seems to be missing in BRS. Guyton is a much easier read than NMS Physiology, but way much, much longer. Warning: some sections can be very painful to read.

Kaplan Lecture Notes - Section on Physiology

Very good coverage of physiology, although like BRS physiology, a bit weak on coverage of pathophysiology. May occasionally need to supplement from NMS or texts like Guyton or Ganong.

Physiology by Guyton

Great coverage of Physiology and Pathophysiology. Its a very easy read but very long. If you are weak on physio and pathophysio, may be worth the investment to read through Guyton.

Physiology by Ganong

Coverage relatively the same as Guyton. But personally, I prefer Guyton to Ganong because Guyton seems to be an easier read.

First Aid - Section on Physiology

As with all thing First Aid, use only for high yield review last two weeks before exam. Lacks enough details for a comprehensive review of physiology. Never use alone. ■

CHAPTER 56
WHAT TO STUDY IN PHYSIOLOGY

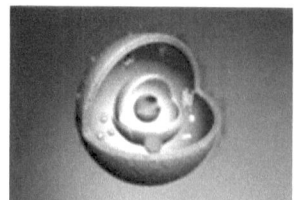

Physiology is one of the minor subjects, but its importance lies in the fact it's the basis for understanding pathophysiology which comprises a really big part of Step 1. You need to study enough of physiology so you understand pathophysiology. Pure physiology is not important, but physiology related to pathophysiology is.

Therefore it is important that you cover this subject well. A lot of times, poor performance in pathophysiology can be traced to inadequate understanding of physiology. Even though physiology is a minor subject, it can impact your overall performance if you don't study it well.

It is fairly obvious that you need to study all physiology that is important or related to pathophysiology. In fact you need to integrate them into pathology primarily. Plus, not all pathophysiology is discussed in pathology. Acid base disorders, spirometric abnormalities, a lot of endocrine physiology, like menstrual and pregnancy related physiology are not found in pathology but rather in physiology. Therefore you need to really cover them properly here.

Cell physiology is important because it's one of the molecular biology topics. And taking some time to study it can help boost your scores.

It is impossible to list down everything you need to study here, so you need to use the guide above to decide on what you need to study on. An alternative is to use the notes on Physiology or an equivalent reviewer which contains what I or other authors think will come out in the exam. ■

CHAPTER 57

FIRST REVISION OF PHYSIOLOGY

How to Study Physiology

Physiology is mostly made up of processes you need to understand. Although some item lists do occur, it's still mostly processes. Understand that what underlies most pathology is a disruption of these physiologic processes and that the basis of most drugs is the restoration of the function of these physiologic processes.

The books we will be using in the course will either be my notes on Physiology or BRS Physiology. We use Guyton as a reference book in case we don't understand a particular topic very well.

The purpose of the first revision is to memorize the topics and insure you know them. You also need to integrate the various systems in physiology together.

Memorize Headings and Subheadings

First, you need to organize the different topics in physiology in your head. You can do this by memorizing the headings and subheadings for each chapter first. Then tackle the details. Physiology is organized by system and the different physiologic process under each system.

An alternative, especially if you are integrating anatomy, physiology and biochemistry to pathology, and then physiology and biochemistry to pharmacology is to memorize the pathology headings and subheadings and just file the physiologic concepts associated with each pathology under the headings and subheadings of pathology.

For example, you integrate anatomy of the heart and cardiovascular system to physiology of the cardiovascular system. Then you integrate them to cardiovascular pathology, understanding what anatomic structure or physiologic process is disrupted by the pathology. Then you integrate everything into cardiovascular pharmacology. Understanding what drugs work on certain pathology and the anatomic structure or physiologic process the drugs tries to affect to restore function and repair the pathology.

Studying this way files the contents under pathology headings and subheadings rather than on physiology headings. This can make the information you need to retain more compact and integrated together.

Memorizing Lists of Concepts

Although most of what you will study in physiology are processes, there are some lists that you need to memorize. When memorizing list of items, the first step is to memorize each item without going through the details of each item. Once you start going through the details of each item make sure you know the differences between the items in the list and not just memorize the characteristics of the items.

For example, we want to memorize the factors that control arterial pressures. You first memorize that there are three, (1) Baroreceptor response, (2) CNS, (3) ANS. so if someone asks what factors control arterial pressure and you can enumerate all three without reading, you have got it. Next thing you need to do is to understand how these three control centers differ in the way they control arterial pressure. I can't discuss everything in detail, but a simple way to differentiate the three is this way. Baroreceptors are located in the carotid and provide information about blood pressure to the CNS. The CNS has their own receptors too and control blood pressure by acting either directly on the heart or on the blood vessels. The ANS meanwhile act mostly on the peripheral system either through reflex mechanisms directly to the heart or blood vessels or relay impulses from the CNS to the cardiovascular system.

When you go through the details of the baroreceptor response, you are now dealing with a process you need to memorize. We will discuss that in detail in the next section. Going through the details of CNS control, we are faced with another list. So we memorize that list. CNS control of arterial pressure is mediated in three areas, (1) Medulla, (2) Hypothalamus, and (3) Cortex. Now differentiate the three. Medullary control exerted through two mechanism: Pressor system and depressor system that acts on the blood vessel by activating or withdrawing vasoconstrictor influence. And secondly on a cardioaccelerator and cardioinhibitory center that acts on the sympathetic and vagus nerve to the heart. The hypothalamus is where temperature changes and emotional stress influence arterial pressure. It acts through the medullary centers. The cortex mediates biofeedback and the fight or flight response and they influence arterial pressure via the other centers.

Details of the ANS control invariably lead to a list of two namely the parasympathetic and sympathetic system. Study the difference between the two in terms of function (vasodilator vs. vasoconstrictor, cardioinhibitory vs, cardioaccelerator), location, receptor, mediator, etc.

Memorizing Processes

Most of what you need to memorize in physiology will be processes. In fact understanding and mastering these physiologic processes will a lot of times help you understand pathology and pharmacology better. As a review, when memorizing process the first step is to memorize the steps. Once you can enumerate the steps, you start studying the details of each step. Understand what happens on each step. Then relate them to the other steps in the process. A step could produce something, modify something, etc. How do they affect other steps in the same process or in other processes? What happens when this step is disrupted, speeds up or modified? These will help you understand the process better and provides a point to integrate with pathology and pharmacology later.

We will continue with the example earlier with baroreceptor response. Memorize the steps in the process of which there are three. (1) baroreceptor generates receptor potential in response to pressure, (2) receptor potential generates action potential that travels through two nerves, aortic and sinus nerves (3) causes reflex slowing of the heart via the vagus nerve and withdrawal of sympathetic tone to blood vessel. This is known as the baroreceptor or moderator reflex. We can actually go to deeper levels. For example, how pressure in the vessel wall generates receptor potential is another process. Action potential passes through the aortic and sinus nerves, results in a list of 2 and you need to describe the difference (sinus nerve more sensitive than aortic nerve).

We then need to know what happens when each step are disrupted or modified. For example, you can increase the pressure on the receptors by massaging the carotids. What will happen then? What if there is an increased sensitivity in the baroreceptor system like in Stokes-Adams in elderly individual? And so on and so forth.

Integrating the Different Systems in Physiology

Physiology is divided into systems. And we study each system and the physiologic processes that occur under each system. But we must understand that this system do not operate independent of each other. They affect each other. A problem in the cardiovascular system can cause problems in the renal system and vice versa, because they are interconnected. When you encounter such interconnection, it is best to integrate them.

What do we mean by integrating them? For example when you first go through the ANS, it discusses all organ systems affected by it. When you go through the cardiovascular system, every time any part of the CVS is affected by the ANS, you will encounter a short discussion of the ANS. you can opt to stop there, or you can go and reread the ANS section that discussed the particular topic. The reason you want to reread that topic is to strengthen your integration to the topic. If you just read the short discussion posted in the CVS discussion, you will not be integrating the two topics completely. But only partially. Come exam time, when the question requires you to do a full integration instead of a partial one in order to come up with the answer, you run the risk of missing the answer or taking too much time in the process.

Reviewing Concepts from Different Contexts

There is a need to review concepts in the different context in which they are presented to us. The reason is that the USMLE can ask the questions based on any context. If you study the concept in only one context and then the question presents the concept in a different context, you need to analyze and think through the concept to understand it from the other context before you can answer the question. That takes more time and you need every second you have for the USMLE.

Second is that by reviewing concepts from different context, you not only study the concept again, you increase the total number of relationships between concepts. You are increasing your retention of those concepts by using the principle of relation and repetition.

For example, the autonomic nervous system. When you first study the ANS, you look at it from the point of view of the ANS and how they related to each individual system they affect. However, as you study each individual system, say cardiovascular system or gastrointestinal system, you again encounter the ANS in relation to their function within the CVS or GIS respectively. You can opt to skip the discussion on

ANS in each of these systems as you have studied them when you studied the ANS as a whole. But it's better for you to study them again in the context of each system because the questions can be in the context of the CVS or GIS even though we are talking about the ANS.

If you study it in the context of the ANS alone, when it's a CVS question and you have to recall the ANS in relation to CVS, your thought process has to go through the ANS, then drill down to ANS related to CVS. This will take you a few seconds longer to answer the question. It may not seem much, but if every question takes you 15 seconds longer to answer because you have to take this extra analytic step during the exam, 20 questions and you lose 5 minutes. 40 questions and you lose 10 minutes. You can use those extra minutes analyzing tougher questions and giving yourself a better chance of scoring higher.

Answering Chapter by Chapter Quiz in BRS Physiology

It is important to understand the importance of monitoring whether you are making progress or not. Progress in this case is not how much you have read, but how much information you have retained and whether you can recall them. There are only two ways to do this, either by answering questions or using flashcards. At this stage, we use questions.

It is best to test yourself after you finish each chapter in order to know if you have understood enough, retained enough and be able to recall enough before going to the next chapter. This tests that you have actually made progress. For Physiology, we are currently using the end of chapter quiz in BRS Physiology for this purpose. If you get any question wrong reread the full section in the appropriate chapter.

Reading up from Guyton or Ganong on Topics You Find Hard to Understand

Invariably, you will encounter some concepts you do not understand. Reviewers are written for compactness and easy review, they presume you already know all the topics. Therefore, you may need to occasionally refer to textbooks to clarify any topic you have not understood well. In physiology, the texts we use can either be Guyton or Ganong. If you had a formal learning phase, then chances are you will spend less time referring to textbooks. If you did not, then you may find yourself going to textbooks more often. ■

CHAPTER 58

SECOND REVISION OF PHYSIOLOGY

Continue to Memorize All Topics Covered in First Revision

The main purpose of the second revision is to try to integrate related topics between different subjects together. For physiology, this includes anatomy, pathology and pharmacology.

For the second revision, you should continue memorizing what you have studied in the first revision. The purpose is to cement what you have memorized in the first revision. Don't just read through them; try to recite them out loud without looking at them.

Integrate Anatomy and Physiology

At this stage of your review, you should try to integrate anatomy and physiology together. Integrating anatomy to physiology means correlating structure and function in order to understand how organ systems work. For example, how does the structure of the lungs contribute to its function for gas exchange? The gross anatomy of the thorax and lungs are optimized for ventilations while the microscopic anatomy(histology) is optimized for gas exchange between the environment and blood. The structure of the nephron is optimized to regulate water and electrolyte excretion by the body. The glomerulus is optimized to filter the necessary elements and the anatomy of the tubules is optimized to promote the proper osmotic gradient for controlling water exchange. Understanding this structure and function correlation will help you understand pathology and pharmacology better.

You can write the result of your integration into the margins of the notes you are using so it is easier to review them in later revisions without having to do the integration again.

Integrate Anatomy and Physiology into Pathology

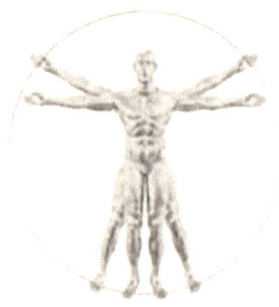

The next step is to integrate into pathology. By studying a specific process properly, you can integrate it into pathology much more easily and understand what is actually happening in the pathologic process. Again, we will use the nephron as an example.

We can look at the nephron as a process by which urine is formed in order to regulate body fluids and electrolyte content. The steps are (1) Proximal Convoluted Tubule, (2) Thin Loop of Henle, (3) Thick Loop of Henle, (4) Distal Convoluted Tubule, (5) Cortical Collecting Tunule, (6) Medullary Collecting Duct. Each step of the process does different things. The PCT reabsorbs everything in various proportion. Thin loop of

Henle reabsorbs water primarily but much less than PCT. Thick Loop reabsorbs Na and K primarily but again less than PCT. The DCT reabsorbs Na, Cl and Ca. The CCT reabsorbs Na and Water in exchange for K and reabsorbs K in exchange for H. Therefore, if there is a lack of Na, K or water in the body, urine becomes acidic. The MCD reabsorbs Na and Water in response to Antidiuretic Hormone.

Once you understand what each steps do, you know that any pathology in any part of the nephron will cause specific problems. Lack of ADH will cause diuresis. Unresponsiveness of Collecting Duct cells to ADH will also cause diuresis. Various RTA's or Renal Tubular Acidosis are caused by dysfunction in the tubules. Type 1 is due to distal tubule defect. There is failure to reabsorb K in exchange for H causing acidosis and hypokalemia due to loss of K in the urine and accumulation of H in the blood. Type 2 has pathology in the PCT. Defect due to inability to reabsorb bicarbonate. This leads to acidosis, but not hypokalemia since the CCT is functioning normally and exchanging K for H. This is also why the acidosis is not as severe as Type 1 and the urine in type 2 can be acidified to less than pH of 5.3. Type 2 can be an isolated defect or a more generalized form that affects all of PCT function leading to phosphaturia, glycosuria, aminoaciduria, etc.

Therefore by outlining first the process, than filling in where in the process the pathology takes place, it is much easier to understand the dysfunction caused by the pathology and how they differ from each other as the above example illustrates.

Integrate Physiology into Pharmacology

We now need to integrate physiology into pharmacology. Again, by studying the physiologic process properly, we can integrate physiology into pharmacology more easily and understand the mechanism of drug action and the various effects it will have on the process itself. We will continue to use the nephron as an example.

When we integrated physiology into pathology, it was enough for us to know what electrolytes and substrates are absorbed and excreted in the different parts of the body. However, in order to properly integrate physiology, we need to understand the exact process that is responsible for excreting or reabsorbing these electrolytes and substrates. We can't possibly discuss in detail all the processes involved in the absorption and excretion of the different electrolytes and substrates in the different parts of the tubule. You can read that in my Physiology notes. For this discussion, we will use the processes in the Loop of Henle as an example.

The main process occurring in the Loop of Henle is the Na-K-Cl co-transporter that drives these 3 electrolytes from the lumen into the cell. A Na-K pump on the basal part of the cell pumps sodium out into the interstium and K into the cell. This keeps Na in the cell low and creates a gradient that drives Na into the cell through the co-transporter. Cl flows out through a Cl channel into the systemic circulation. With both pumps pumping K into the cell, the K is flowing to the lumen through its concentration gradient. This brings with it an excess positive charge which drives Ca and Mg from the lumen to the systemic circulation.

Drugs that affect the tubules usually cause diuresis. Diuretics act on these transporters to cause their effect. Roughly all diuretics can be divided into those that affect primarily water excretion and those that affect Na excretion. Those that affect water excretion are the ADH agonists and antagonists affecting primarily the collecting duct. Those that affect Na excretion include carbonic anhydrase inhibitors that affect PCT, loop diuretics that affect Loop of Henle, Thiazides that affect DCT and the K-sparing diuretics that affect the CCT. Osmotic diuretics affect both Na and water excretion.

For example, loop diuretics act primarily on the Na-Cl-K co transporter. The effect is that NaCl is not reabsorbed. This causes a massive NaCl diuresis. The diluting ability of the nephron is reduced because the loop of Henle is responsible for significant dilution of the urine. Significant Ca can also be loss due to loss of the positive charge from K. The presence of a large amount of Na to the CCT can cause hypokalemia as the K is exchanged for Na. The massive K in the urine caused by this exchange can cause secretion of protons in exchange for K. This leads to hypokalemic alkalosis.

Of course, you need to know more details of the loop diuretics in pharmacology than what was presented. But by understanding physiologic process and integrating them into pharmacology, you can gain a better understanding of the effects of the drugs and potential side effect.

Usually when you go through pathology or pharmacology, there is a brief discussion integrating them to relevant topics in physiology or biochemistry. However, these discussions are brief and the integration is not thorough. It is up to you to go into a more detailed integration to cement your knowledge. Plus the integration is done piecemeal and does not give you a broad picture. Sometimes, the only way you can answer some of the questions that appear in the USMLE is to see the big integrated picture.

Use Physiology Flashcards

At this point you can start using physiology flashcards to increase your ability to recall the concepts better and faster. You can use Askdoc's High Yield Flashcard Review for Physiology or make your own using the topics in my notes or BRS Physiology

Use Study Notes and Outline Notes Primarily

If you are using my notes, then use the notes only. By this time you should not be referring to textbooks if you did your first revision correctly. You should have corrected any deficiency of the learning phase and covered any topics you did not understand in the first revision.

Make use of the outline notes primarily, trying to remember the details and only glancing at the study notes if you can't recall all the details. This will help cement your retention of the materials.

If you are using BRS Physiology or other books. Then try to read the headings and subheadings in bold print and try to recall the details. Glance at the details only if you can't remember them.

Use Per Subject Quiz like Kaplan Q Book

For the second revision, test your mastery of physiology by using per subject quiz like Kaplan Q book. Aim for at least 80% or higher. ■

CHAPTER 59

THIRD REVISION OF PHYSIOLOGY

Continue Memorizing all Topics Covered in First Revision

For the third revision, the main purpose is to cover your weak points. At this stage you are doing online Q Banks already as part of your Test Preparation Phase. You use it also to spot weak points and cover them.

You need to continue to memorize all the topics you covered in the first revision. Again, don't just read through them, try to recite them out loud without reading your notes. This will improve your retention and recall of the topics.

Continue Memorizing Integrated Topics you Wrote in Your Notes

It is also very important to continue memorizing the integrated topics you covered in your second revision. You should have written these integrated topics in the margins of your notes so you can refer to them without having to read through everything all over again.

Use Outline Notes Primarily and Try to Recall Details in Study Notes without Reading It

Just like on your second revision, use the outline notes primarily, trying to recall what is in the study notes without looking at them. This will improve your retention of what you have studied. If you are using BRS or other reviewers, then look at the headings and subheadings only and try to recall the details without reading them.

Continue Using Physiology Flashcards

You should continue to improve your retention of what you have studied and improve your ability to recall them randomly. Continue using flashcards for this purpose.

Use Online Q Banks to Determine What Weak Points need to be Covered

At this point in your revision, you should be doing online qbanks as part of your test preparation phase. Use the results of the q bank to pinpoint your weak areas. Study your weak areas one more time. You still cover everything you studied before at least once. But try to go through your weak point's one extra round.

Watch out for integrated topic that you failed to cover in your second revision. Usually a lot of questions in the q bank cover integrated topics. If you discover any new integrated topic in the q bank that you have not studied before, don't just study the answers to the question, go back and cover the integrated topic through your notes. The reason is most integrated topic has multiple points that need to be integrated. An integrated topic question in the qbank may cover only one point of let's say 10 points of that topic. If you just study the question, you know only 1 point and not 10. If an actual question on that topic comes out in the actual exam, it may be based on a different point of the same concept, which you did not cover. ■

CHAPTER 60

HIGH YIELD REVIEW OF PHYSIOLOGY

High Yield Review is very different from the standard prep you just went through. In high yield review, you concentrate on covering only the highest yield material that will come out in the exam. At this stage you have finished your standard prep which means you have basically covered both high yield and low yield material in Physiology. What we want to do now is make sure that what you remember best is the highest yield information.

For this high yield review, your choice of study material include my outline notes on Physiology, First Aid for the USMLE Step 1 - Section on Physiology or Askdoc's High Yield Flashcard Review for Physiology. You should be doing this the last two weeks before you sit for the examination.

The best combination is to read through my outline notes in physiology. Then go through the flashcards for quick recall exercise. ∎

***

unit 9

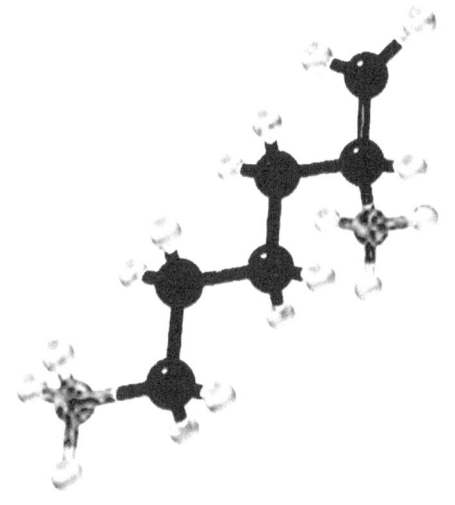

How to Review
Biochemistry

CHAPTER 61
INTRODUCTION

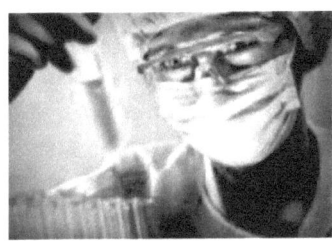

Biochemistry is considered one of the minor subjects. But its importance is inflated because you need a very good understanding of biochemistry to do well in Pathology and Pharmacology, two of the most important subject in Step 1.

One of the most important things you have to know about biochemistry is that most of it involves processes. Although physiology also involves a lot of processes, the main difference is that while all the steps in physiologic processes is more or less important, in biochemical processes, only key steps are important. You must emphasize in your study the understanding of how this processes works and that disruption of the steps in the processes can result in pathology. ■

CHAPTER 62
STUDY MATERIALS FOR BIOCHEMISTRY

Study materials for biochemistry can be divided into texts, reviewers, flash cards and q banks.

Textbooks - none

Reviewers include

- Askdoc's Biochemistry Notes - Study Notes, Outline Notes, Summary Notes
- Lippincott's Illustrated Review of Biochemistry
- Kaplan's Lecture Notes - Section on Biochemistry
- NMS Biochemistry
- NMS Genetics
- First Aid - Section on Biochemistry and Genetics

Flashcards include

- Askdoc's High Yield Flashcards for Biochemistry

Q banks include

- Kaplan's Q Book - Section on Biochemistry
- Kaplan's Online Q Bank - Section on Biochemistry
- USMLE World Online Q Bank - Section on Biochemistry

We will discuss the more important study materials in more detail.

Askdoc's Notes on Biochemistry - Study Notes, Outline Notes, Summary Notes

Askdoc's Notes on Biochemistry are the recommended

study material for the course. The notes follow all the study methodologies and principles of learning taught in the course. The Study Notes cover all the topics that will be tested in the exam. It covers both low yield and high yield topics. The Outline Notes cover the high yield topics for high yield review. The Summary Notes contain instructions and explanations on how to study each chapter properly.

Lippincott's Illustrated Review of Biochemistry

This is a very good introductory book on Biochemistry. If you are an old grad like me and you have forgotten most of your biochemistry and the little you remember is obsolete, this is a very good book to start your review on. However, there is very minimal discussion of genetics. Another plus is that a lot of topics are integrated with Lippincott's Illustrated Review of Pharmacology.

Kaplan's Lecture Notes - Section on Biochemistry and Genetics

Found this to be the best in terms of coverage of all the Kaplan lecture notes. Superb coverage of Biochemistry and Genetics. If you are an old grad, however, you may find it to understand. In my case I used Lippincott's first before using this book. Very good coverage of Molecular Biology topics too. Use as main reviewer.

NMS Biochemistry

Good book on Biochemistry but inferior to Lippincott over all. Stronger coverage of Genetics than Lippincott. Weaker in both biochemistry and genetics than Kaplan.

NMS Genetics

Very good coverage of genetics. However, it covers too many topics not tested on the board but needed to understand the more advanced concepts that are tested on the board. So if you are an old grad and forgot your genetics, you can use this book to catch up.

First Aid - Section on Biochemistry and Genetics

First Aid for the USMLE Step 1 is only good for high yield review done a week or two before the exam. Otherwise, there is too little information in the book for a comprehensive review Biochemistry. You need to do a comprehensive review if you want to do well. More so if you are an IMG. ■

CHAPTER 63
WHAT TO STUDY FOR BIOCHEMISTRY

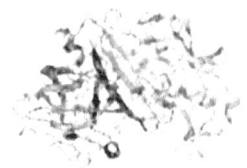

Biochemistry is one of the minor subjects. Its importance lies in the fact that biochemical processes underlie our understanding of pathologic processes as well as mechanism of actions of drugs. Therefore, it is important to study them well.

You will need to concentrate on key steps. Unlike in physiology, where every step of a process in important, most steps in biochemistry are intermediate steps. Key steps are important steps. They are either rate-limiting steps, or steps where positive or negative feedbacks occur. They could also be steps where some important by-product or substrate is produced or modified.

Since its main importance is in the understanding of pharmacology and pathology, it is fairly obvious that you need to concentrate on integrating biochemistry into those subjects. Metabolism and genetics underlie most of the systems in the human body.

A lot of molecular biology can be found in biochemistry,

especially in genetics, where it's called molecular genetics. Molecular genetics is the basis for our understanding of how a lot of diseases occur and could be the basis of finding cures. Hence it's importance in pathology and pharmacology.

We cannot list here everything that you need to study in biochemistry but you can use the guidelines above to decide what you need to study. Or you can use my notes on biochemistry or other reviewers to know what I or other authors think will come out in the exam. ■

CHAPTER 64
FIRST REVISION OF BIOCHEMISTRY

How to Study Biochemistry

Biochemistry is composed mostly of processes that you need to memorize. They are mostly metabolic processes that occur within cells. Unlike physiologic processes, most biochemical processes have key steps and intermediate steps. You need to know the key steps very well, while you just need to know where the intermediate steps are located in the process. Key steps are usually rate-limiting steps, site of negative or positive feedback and where substrate or energy is produced.

Memorize Headings and Subheadings

First, you need to organize the different topics in Biochemistry in your head so that you have a general framework to retain and recall the information you need for the examination. Biochemistry can be divided into metabolism and genetics. Alternatively, file them under pathology topics when you integrate biochemistry into pathology.

Memorizing List of Concepts

In memorizing lists, it is important to memorize first the list of items before tackling the individual items in detail. After you have gone through the details of each item, try to determine how the items differ from each other so it's easy to differentiate them from each other when questions are asked.

For example, the secondary structures of proteins are composed of five configurations. The first step is to memorize all five. (1) alpha-helix, (2) beta-sheet, (3) beta bends, (4) non-repetitive structure and (5) super secondary structure or motifs. After you have memorized all five and can recite them out loud. The next step is to memorize the details. For example details of the alpha helix include hydrogen bonds, number of amino acids per turns, and amino acids that can disrupt the helix. There is too much details to discuss here so refer to the appropriate reviewer as needed.

Once you have gone through the details of all 5 secondary structure, the next step is to make sure you know the difference between all five. It's not enough to know there is a difference; you need to know exactly what makes them different from each other. Of course the alpha helix form helices and not all the peptide bonds are involved in hydrogen bonding. Beta sheets form pleated sheets and all peptide bonds from hydrogen bonds. And so on and so forth.

Memorizing Processes

In memorizing processes, it is best to first memorize the steps, then memorize details of each step, then memorize what happens when certain steps are modified. For example, the citric acid cycle is composed of a series of steps with the endpoint of producing two-thirds of the ATP in humans. The way to tackle this process is first to memorize the steps. Then take note of where ATP is produced and other substrate. Then study in detail each step of the process. Then finally play what ifs with modifications of the steps.

First, all the steps. (1) Acetyl-CoA from pyruvate, (2) Citrate from oxaloacetate and Acetyl-CoA, (3) Isomerization of citrate to Isocitrate, (4) Isocitrate to alpha-ketoglutarate by oxidation and decarboxylation, (5) Succinyl CoA from alpha-ketoglutarate by oxidative decarboxylation, (6) Cleavage of

Succinyl CoA to form Succinate, (7) Fumarate from oxidation of Succinate, (8) Malate from hydration of fumarate, then (9) oxaloacetate from oxidation of malate.

Once you have memorized all the steps, you now take note of all areas where ATP is produced. ATP is produced in the Electron Transport Chain by the oxidation of NADH and FADH2. Oxidation of NADH produces 3 ATP while oxidation of FADH2 produces 2 ATP. The citric acid cycle produces 3 NADH and one FADH2. The 3 NADH is produced from oxidative decarboxylation of Isocitrate to alpha-ketoglutarate, alpha-ketoglutarate to Succinyl CoA and oxidation of malate to oxaloacetate. FADH2 is produced from oxidation of succinate to fumarate. There is also a substrate level phosphorylation when succinyl Co A is cleaved to form succinate. Also take note of where CO2 is formed as well as total ATP produced.

The next step is to study each reaction in detail, which includes the enzymes catalyzed by the reaction, all the reactive substances and byproducts. Once that is done, study and memorize the regulatory steps that activate and inhibit the cycle. Later on when you study some pathology that can affect the citric acid cycle, e.g. lack of O2 or ADP for example, you can understand better what happens.

There is a systematic way of studying processes that will not only help you remember them better, but even anticipate possible questions that will come out in the exam.

Integrating Metabolism

Although the metabolism of each substrate is discussed individually, we need to understand there are many metabolic processes that interact with each other. Metabolism of proteins, carbohydrates and fats influence each other and there are common pathways through which their metabolism interacts. Therefore it is important to connect metabolism into a whole picture after studying them individually.

Answering per Chapter Quiz in Lippincott's Illustrated Review of Biochemistry

It is important to understand the importance of monitoring whether you are making progress or not. Progress in this case is not how much you have read, but how much information you have retained and whether you can recall them. There are only two ways to do this, either by answering questions or using flashcards. At this stage, we use questions.

It is best to test yourself after you finish each chapter in order to know if you have understood enough, retained enough and be able to recall enough before going to the next chapter. This tests that you have actually made progress. For Biochemistry, we are currently using the end of chapter quiz in Lippincott's Biochemistry for this purpose. If you get any question wrong reread the full section in the appropriate chapter.

Reading up from Lippincott's Illustrated Review of Biochemistry on Topics You Find Hard to Understand

Unless you did a formal learning phase, there might be some topics that you did not understand very well during your first revision. In that case, you need to read up the topics in a basic text. Although Lippincott's Illustrated Review can be considered a reviewer, it has basic discussions on all the major topics and is fairly easy to understand. ■

CHAPTER 65

SECOND REVISION OF BIOCHEMISTRY

Continue to Memorize All Topics Covered in First Revision

The main purpose of the second revision is to try to integrate related topics between different subjects together. For biochemistry, this includes anatomy, physiology, pharmacology and pathology.

For the second revision, you should continue memorizing what you have studied in the first revision. The purpose is to cement what you have memorized in the first revision. Don't just read through them; try to recite them out loud without looking at them.

Integrate Anatomy and Physiology into Biochemistry

After you have integrated structure and function through anatomy and physiology, integrate relevant topics in biochemistry into them. For example, the hormone insulin and glucagon has a very big role in metabolism of carbohydrates proteins and fat. Hormones are discussed in more detail in physiology, while the metabolism they control is discussed in more detail in biochemistry. Hence the need to integrate that knowledge into a whole concept.

Integrate Biochemistry into Pathology and Pharmacology

A lot of pathology is based on disruptions of a biochemical process; therefore it is important to integrate the biochemical processes. For an example, refer to the section on How to Study Pathology, which discussed integrating arachidonic acid metabolism, a biochemical process to pathology and pharmacology.

Use Biochemistry Flashcards

At this point you can start using pharmacology flashcards to increase your ability to recall the concepts better and faster. You can use Askdoc's High Yield Flashcard Review for Biochemistry or make your own using the topics in my notes or from Lippincott's.

Use Only Study Notes and Outline Notes

If you are using my notes, then use the notes only. By this time you should not be referring to textbooks if you did your first revision correctly. You should have corrected any deficiency of the learning phase and covered any topics you did not understand in the first revision.

Make use of the outline notes primarily, trying to remember the details and only glancing at the study notes if you can't recall all the details. This will help cement your retention of the materials.

If you are using Lippincott's or other books, then try to read the headings and subheadings in bold print and try to recall the details. Glance at the details only if you can't remember them.

Use Per Subject Quiz like Kaplan Q Book

For the second revision, test your mastery of

pharmacology by using per subject quiz like Kaplan Q book. Aim for at least 80% or higher. ■

CHAPTER 66

THIRD REVISION OF BIOCHEMISTRY

Continue Memorizing all Topics Covered in First Revision

For the third revision, the main purpose is to cover your weak points. At this stage you are doing online Q Banks already as part of your Test Preparation Phase. You use it also to spot weak points and cover them.

You need to continue to memorize all the topics you covered in the first revision. Again, don't just read through them, try to recite them out loud without reading your notes. This will improve your retention and recall of the topics.

Continue Memorizing Integrated Topics you Wrote in Your Notes

It is also very important to continue memorizing the integrated topics you covered in your second revision. You should have written these integrated topics in the margins of your notes so you can refer to them without having to read through everything all over again.

Use Outline Notes Primarily and Try to Recall Details in Study Notes without Reading It

Just like on your second revision, use the outline notes primarily, trying to recall what is in the study notes without looking at them. This will improve your retention of what you have studied. If you are using Lippincott's or other reviewers, then look at the headings and subheadings only and try to recall the details without reading them.

Continue Using Biochemistry Flashcards

You should continue to improve your retention of what you have studied and improve your ability to recall them randomly. Continue using flashcards for this purpose.

Use Online Q Banks to Determine What Weak Points need to be Covered

At this point in your revision, you should be doing online qbanks as part of your test preparation phase. Use the results of the q bank to pinpoint your weak areas. Study your weak areas one more time. You still cover everything you studied before at least once. But try to go through your weak points one extra round.

Watch out for integrated topic that you failed to cover in your second revision. Usually a lot of questions in the q bank cover integrated topics. If you discover any new integrated topic in the q bank that you have not studied before, don't just study the answers to the question, go back and cover the integrated topic through your notes. The reason is most integrated topics have multiple points that need to be integrated. An integrated topic question in the qbank may cover only one point of let's say 10 points of that topic. If you just study the question, you know only 1 point and not 10. If an actual question on that topic comes out in the actual exam, it may be based on a different point of the same concept, which you did not cover. ■

299

CHAPTER 67

HIGH YIELD REVIEW OF BIOCHEMISTRY

High Yield Review is very different from the standard prep you just went through. In high yield review, you concentrate on covering only the highest yield material that will come out in the exam. At this stage you have finished your standard prep which means you have basically covered both high yield and low yield material in Biochemistry. What we want to do now is make sure that what you remember best are the highest yield information.

For this high yield review, your choice of study material include my outline notes on Biochemistry, First Aid for the USMLE Step 1 - Section on Biochemistry or Askdoc's High Yield Flashcard Review for Biochemistry. You should be doing this the last two weeks before you sit for the examination.

The best combination is to read through my outline notes in biochemistry. Then go through the flashcards for a quick recall exercise. ■

***

unit 10

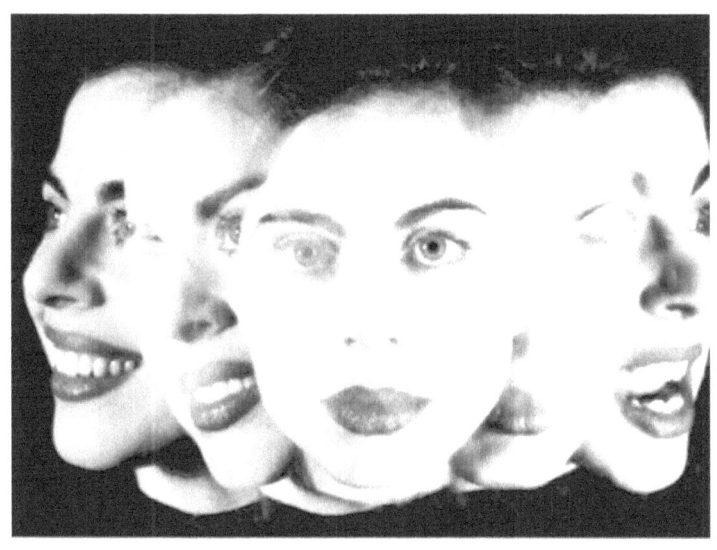

HOW TO REVIEW
BEHAVIORAL SCIENCES

CHAPTER 68
INTRODUCTION

For American Medical Students, Behavioral Science is probably the easiest part of Step 1. They don't really have to study that much. But for a lot of IMG's (International Medical Graduate), it is a very hard subject. The main reason is that half of behavioral science is medical ethics and law and that is culture based. Therefore, if the IMG's country of origin has a culture that is very different from the United States, it's not easy to answer questions that are culturally based.

The other half of Behavioral Sciences covers Biostatistics and Epidemiology, Life Cycle and Human Development, Psychology and Psychiatry and the Practice of Medicine in the US. The IMG usually do not find this part much of a problem. ■

CHAPTER 69
STUDY MATERIALS FOR BEHAVIORAL SCIENCES

Study materials for behavioral sciences can be divided into texts, reviewers, flash cards and q banks.

Textbooks - none
Reviewers include
- Askdoc's Behavioral Sciences Notes - Study Notes, Outline Notes, Summary Notes
- Kaplan's Lecture Notes - Section on Behavioral Sciences
- BRS Behavioral Sciences
- NMS Behavioral Sciences
- First Aid - Section on Behavioral Sciences

Flashcards include
- Askdoc's High Yield Behavioral Sciences Flashcards

Q banks include
- Kaplan's Q Book - Section on Behavioral Sciences
- Kaplan's Online Q Bank - Section on Behavioral Sciences
- USMLE World Online Q Bank - Section on Behavioral Sciences
- We will discuss the more important study materials in more detail.

Askdoc's Notes on Behavioral Sciences -

Study Notes, Outline Notes and Summary Notes

Askdoc's Notes on Behavioral Sciences are the recommended study material for the course. The notes follow all the study methodologies and principles of learning taught in the course. The Study Notes cover all the topics that will be tested in the exam. It covers both low yield and high yield topics. The Outline Notes cover the high yield topics for high yield review. The Summary Notes contain instructions and explanations on how to study each chapter properly.

Kaplan Lecture Notes - Section on Behavioral Sciences

Good coverage of BS topics, but not as good as BRS. The best thing about Kaplan is that it has a list of *Do's and Dont's* on Medical Ethics and Law. Use that as a guide on how to answer questions on those topics. It is still best to study Medical Ethics and Law using case-based examples in the online q bank.

BRS Behavioral Sciences

Very good coverage of BS topics. All you need to do well in Behavioral Sciences except on questions about Medical Ethics and Law. Use Kaplan and the online Q banks for that.

NMS Behavioral Science

What can I say, not really very good.

First Aid - Section on Behavioral Sciences

As with all things First Aid, use only as high yield review about two weeks before the exam. Inadequate for comprehensive review. Never use alone.

CHAPTER 70

WHAT TO STUDY FOR BEHAVIORAL SCIENCES

Although behavioral science is considered one of the minor four, in reality it comprises 12 to 15% of the exam. Almost as big as Pharmacology or Microbiology and Immunology. However, half of behavioral sciences will be questions about medical ethics and law. And most of the cases are culture based. Therefore, they are hard to learn. The other half, however, like biostatistics, psychology, etc. are easy to learn and memorize.

Medical ethics and law are best learned using the case method, so you can see how they apply in particular situations, therefore, you make use of the online q banks to practice how to answer those questions. ∎

CHAPTER 71
FIRST REVISION OF BEHAVIORAL SCIENCES

How to Study Behavioral Sciences

Behavioral Sciences review can basically be divided into two parts. The first part can be studied by memorizing various topics from a reviewer, while the second part should be studied using cases. The first part covers psychology, basic psychiatry, life cycle and human development, biostatistics and epidemiology as well as medical practice in the US. The second part involves understanding how to make decisions regarding ethics and law. These are studied differently which we will outline below.

How to Study the First Part of Behavioral Sciences

The first part of Behavioral Science covers basic psychology and psychiatry, life cycle and human development, biostatistics and epidemiology and characteristics of medical practice in the US. It's straightforward memorization of facts. There will be some computations in biostatistics but very few probably less than 5 in the whole exam. Epidemiology will cover most common causes of death, mortality rates, etc.

The recommended reviewer for this subject is either Askdoc's notes on Behavioral Sciences or BRS Behavioral

Sciences. Both contain what you need to know about these topics. Most of the things you will study here are list of concepts you need to memorize and almost no process. So make sure you are able to distinguish between concepts not just characterize each concept. An example is when studying the different defense mechanism, don't just memorize the characteristics of each defense mechanism, but take note of how to differentiate them from each other. A lot of questions will revolve around specific case scenarios and patient behavior and you need to state what defense mechanism is being manifested by the patient. Same thing with personality disorders which unless you take the time to differentiate from each other, may look the same superficially. For example what is the difference between paranoid, schizoid and schizotypal personality disorders?

Reviewing Medical Ethics and Law

The second part of Behavioral Sciences is medical ethics and law or what some people will call social questions. These questions are culture based and therefore most IMG's who live outside the US will have problems on this part. The best way to learn to answer these kinds of questions is through cases. The recommended reviewers for this part of Behavioral Sciences is either Askdoc's Behavioral Science Notes or Kaplan Lecture Notes - section on Behavioral Sciences as well as one of the online Q Banks.

First, read through the guidelines on medical ethics and law on either reviewer. Then when answering questions on medical ethics and law which is usually case-based, try to compare it with the listed guidelines in either book to understand how the guidelines apply to a particular case.

Answering per Chapter Quiz in BRS Behavioral Science

After finishing each chapter, make sure you go through the questions and answer them. Try to get at least 90% correct before proceeding to next chapter. If less than 90% correct go back and restudy the chapter. ■

CHAPTER 72

SECOND REVISION OF BEHAVIORAL SCIENCES

Continue to Memorize All Topics Covered in First Revision

For the second revision, just go through the topics you went through as the first revision. You should be able to go through them much faster. Try to memorize, not just read through them. This involves reading the topics out loud without looking at the text or just glancing at them

You can optionally try to integrate the psychiatric drugs you encounter in the psychiatry section to specific details about the drugs in pharmacology and write them in your notes.

Use Behavioral Science Flashcards

At this point, you can start using Behavioral Science Flashcards to improve your ability to recall what you have memorized faster. You can use Askdoc's High Yield Flashcard Review of Behavioral Sciences or make your own using the topics in my notes or in BRS.

Use Per Subject Quiz like Kaplan Q Book

For the second revision, test your mastery of the topic by using Kaplan Q Book. ■

CHAPTER 73

THIRD REVISION OF BEHAVIORAL SCIENCES

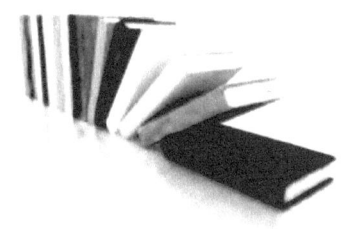

Continue Memorizing all Topics Covered in First and Second Revision

For the third revision, just continue memorizing all the topics you covered in the first and second revision. Continue reviewing the cases for the medical ethics and law part of your review. If you had integrated the psychiatry topics with pharmacology continue to study that.

Use Outline Notes Primarily and Try to Recall Details in Study Notes without Reading It

At this stage, if you are using my Notes, use the outline

notes primarily, recall details in the study notes, and then glance at study noted only if you fail to recall the details. This will help cement your retention of the details and ability to recall them. If you are using BRS, try to read only the headings and sub headings (those in bold print) and recall the details below them.

Continue to Use Behavioral Science Flashcard

At this point you are trying to cement what you know and train yourself to recall all you have studied randomly at will. Using Flashcards will help you do that.

Use Online Q Banks to Determine What Weak Points need to be Covered

At this stage, you have been doing online Q banks for some time already. Use the online Q banks to determine what your weak points are and cover them by reading through the topics you missed. If you miss the answers because you forgot, then just read through them once. If you miss the answer because you understood the topic differently from what the question is pointing out. Take time to reread the whole chapter and try to see if you understood it fully this time. ■

CHAPTER 74

HIGH YIELD REVIEW OF BEHAVIORAL SCIENCES

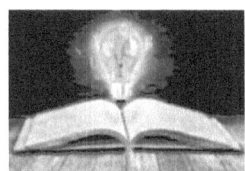

High Yield Review is very different from the standard prep you just went through. In high yield review, you concentrate on covering only the highest yield material that will come out in the exam. At this stage you have finished your standard prep which means you have basically covered both high yield and low yield material in Behavioral Science. What we want to do now is make sure that what you remember best are the highest yield information.

For this high yield review, your choice of study material includes my outline notes on Behavioral Sciences, First Aid for the USMLE Step 1 Behavioral Sciences or Askdoc's High Yield Flashcard Review for Behavioral Sciences. You should be doing this the last two weeks before you sit for the examination. ■

***

unit 11

Test Preparation Phase

CHAPTER 75

INTRODUCTION

Test Preparation Phase is probably one of the most important determinants of how well you do in the USMLE. Whereas, lack of a proper learning phase is the main problem for Old Grads, and lack of proper mastery phase is the most frequent cause of failure, an inadequate test preparation phase is the most common reason why people get a lower score than they otherwise would have.

For most people, test preparation phase is composed only of answering online q banks. This is actually very good as online q banks are probably one of the biggest reasons why people are getting such high scores. But answering questions is just the start of the test preparation phase. There are a lot of other things you need to do maximize your ability to get a higher score.

Then again, although they are becoming fewer now, there are still those who just read through their reviewer and never bother to do online q banks or self-assessment tests. Suffice to say most of them wind up failing the exam or getting low scores.

Aside from answering Q Banks, it is important for you to understand how questions are constructed. There are basic rules that question construction follows, understanding these basic rules can help you understand what can and cannot come out in questions and prepare for them. It will also help narrow to a certain extent the answer choices for most but not all questions. A lot of times I see people choosing answers that are so far off the mark. Understanding basic principles of question construction can help insure that even if you get the wrong answer, the answer is reasonably close to the right answer. Of course that increases the chance that you will get the right answer.

One of the biggest problems most people face in the USMLE Step 1 is being unable to finish all the questions in a block. That can negatively impact your score tremendously. But you will be surprised at how many people do not practice speed building as part of their test preparation phase. Make going thru questions fast a habit and you can increase your chances of getting a good score. ■

CHAPTER 76

IMPORTANCE OF ONLINE Q BANKS

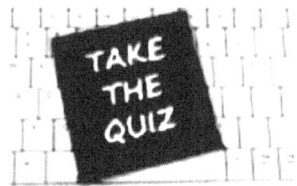

Why Use Online Q Banks

Online Q Banks are probably the number one reason why scores are rising in the USMLE. The reasons are varied and include the following:

It provides a method to assess what you know, so you can pinpoint your weak areas and remedy them. Even if you studied everything multiple times, you won't be strong in all topics. The reason is that we pay more attention to topics we are interested in and tend to ignore what we are not interested in. Even if we read those topics, our mind will tend to wander and just pass through them. So they become weak points. But the USMLE does not care if you are interested in a topic or not. If it's important, it will come out, so you need to cover them.

It lets you get used to answering USMLE type questions which are very different from questions you normally encounter in other exams. There is a certain way the USMLE asks questions that is different from other exams. The reason is that USMLE questions are constructed a certain way. It usually starts with a concept. Then they make the questions harder by rewriting them a certain way. Then the choices are constructed by writing them initially as all correct answers. Then each answer is altered slightly so it becomes the wrong answer until one correct answer remains. Although not all questions go through that process, a lot of them do.

It helps you get used to answering tough questions without going into panic which can be devastating on the actual exam. The first time a lot of people encounter tough USMLE type questions, they are shocked and it impairs overall performance. By going through it before the actual exam, you avoid having this problem on exam day.

It also helps you get used to answering computer based questions and the user interface, so you can concentrate on just doing the exam and not struggle with the user interface. In order to understand the effect of user interface in exam performance, one of my students was scoring in the high 70's in the online Q banks. Suddenly her school wanted her to take an NBME not computer-based but written where you shade a bubble. To make the long story short, she scored poorly although passing. She complained of having difficulty with shading the bubbles. Anyway, she sat for the exam a few weeks later and got a 99/230. So struggling through the computer interface can lower your score.

Comparing Different Q Banks

Now that you know you have to use online q banks for test preparation, which online q banks should you use for your prep? The online Q banks I recommend are the big two, namely Kaplan and USMLE World. I know there are a lot of other new ones out there, but believe me the best is still the big two. Maybe someday, some of the other q banks may make it to my list, but for now I recommend you use the big two.

Questions I am often asked is which is better, Kaplan q banks or USMLE world q banks. To be honest, I find both q banks quite excellent. And you can use either q banks to ace this exam. The main difference is the balance of hard and easy questions between the two. USMLE world has more tough questions although the level of the toughest questions seems to be about equal. However, in terms of mix of tough and easy questions, Kaplan q bank seems closer to the actual exam's mix of tough and easy question.

Another noticeable difference is the fact that Kaplan q banks software tends to balance the difficulty of each block when randomized, while USMLE world can sometimes produce a very tough block and sometimes a very easy one. Of course if you use the filter in Kaplan to select easy and hard questions, you negate this balancing ability in their software.

Each q bank also has a certain way of constructing questions. As you practice with one q bank, you get used to the way the questions are asked and you eventually tend to have an idea on which is the best answer. However, when you switch to the other q bank, you will notice your score falling initially as the way questions are asked is slightly different but after a few blocks, you tend to get back on track in scoring as you get used to it.

So my suggestion is that if you have enough money, use both. Since USMLE World has more tough questions, use that to learn how to answer tough questions. Since Kaplan has a better balance of tough and easy questions, use that to simulate the exam conditions. If you will only be using one qbank either will do. Just make sure to use two thirds of the questions for learning and one third to simulate exam conditions.

Best Way to Use Q Banks

There are a couple of things you need to be aware on how to use q banks properly for your prep.

First, use q banks to learn how to answer tough questions,

not to learn new concepts. The best way to learn concepts and memorize them is in an organized fashion. That is why your medical school teaches medicine that way. If using q banks is the best method, then medical schools should start switching teaching methodologies.

Second, use q banks to pinpoint your weakness and cover them. It is important to know when reading the explanations to answer is enough or you need to re-review a whole section or chapter. If your mistake is centered on lower yield information about a topic or more obscure information, then just read the explanations. But if you are making errors on high yield, core information about a particular topic or it seems you see that you are getting too many questions about a certain topic wrong, and then you may need to go back through the whole section or chapter.

Third, use q banks to simulate actual exam conditions. You need to get used to the way the exam is conducted. It means to work under time pressure and doing multiple blocks consecutively with little or no breaks, so you see how things can go wrong for you when you are under pressure and fix it. The worst part is to find out about them during the exam when it's too late to fix it.

Therefore, it is important that you follow the following guidelines when doing your q banks.

First, use the q banks only once you have done a formal prep. Never use the online q bank as a study tool to learn new facts. Not only is it not very efficient, you also waste the q bank questions. It's like using pliers to hammer in nails. It's possible and I do it once in a while, but it's awkward and not very efficient. Using a hammer is much more efficient. And one more thing, q bank questions cannot be re-used. They lose their effectiveness that way. In the course, students use the online q banks only after they finish their second revision. During first and second revision, they use other q banks to assess their performance.

Second, always do the online q bank on timed, mixed, random, new mode. This simulates the actual conditions during the exam. Other q banks do not allow you to configure questions that way. So make good use of these features since they help you to get used to actual exam conditions.

Third, at the beginning, do only 1 to 2 blocks a day. First, it is expected that when you start q banks, you will be making a lot of mistakes. So for every hour you spent on answering q banks, you need at least two or more hours reviewing the questions you got wrong. Evaluating your thought process and see why you chose the wrong answer. Going through your notes or reviewer again particularly on topics you had a hard time with in the quiz. As you get better, you can do more blocks per day as your mistakes will be less. Second, you need to go slow initially, so you can evaluate your performance, find if anything is wrong and correct it as early as possible. The worst thing that you could do is plough through half the q bank as fast as possible with zero improvement because you did not bother to study your mistakes and learn from them. Remember, the goal is not how many blocks you finish in a given time. The goal is how many blocks you finish with a GOOD score in a given time.

Fourth, don't just review the questions you got wrong but also those you got right but on the following circumstances.

- *It took you a long time to decide the answer.*

- *You know it was a lucky guess.*

- *You were down to last two and got the correct answer*

- *You switch answer at the last minute and got the right answer.*

In these conditions, you don't just study the right answer, but you review your thought process and understand why you almost got the answer wrong. Is it because you misunderstood the questions? You got faked by a small detail in the question.

You have no idea what the question is talking about. You did not know enough details to answer the question. If you know why you erred, you can take steps to correct these errors.

Fifth, take note of integrated topics you encounter in the q banks and make it a point to reread appropriate areas in your notes on integrated topics you missed. The reason you have to do the integration with your notes rather than relying on the q banks explanations is that q bank questions may focus on one point of the whole integrated topic. An integrated topic may have 10 points and you need to cover all 10 points and not just the point emphasized by the q bank question. So when in the actual exam, a different point of the same integrated topic is asked, you can still get the correct answer.

Sixth, make sure you simulate exam conditions at least once using q banks before sitting for the exam. This can help expose ahead of time any problem you may have sitting for the actual exam and correct them.

Seventh, although online q banks can give you a general idea of how prepared you are for the actual exam, only the NBME self-assessment tests are reliable enough to predict your score give or take a few points. ■

CHAPTER 77

CLINICAL VIGNETTES

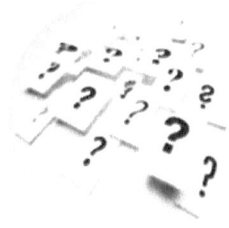

Expect that at least half the questions in the actual USMLE Step 1 will be in the form of clinical vignettes. This is due to the increasing clinical slant of the Steps. The question will not be about clinical medicine. It will focus on a basic medical science principle operating in a particular disease or pathologic condition. However, you need to be able to diagnose the clinical vignette first before you can even begin to answer the question. Even if you know the answer if only it was given to you in a straightforward manner, you will not get partial points for that. So it is important to be able to diagnose as many clinical vignettes correctly as you can.

We have discussed elsewhere on how to train yourself to diagnose clinical vignettes. We also discussed the fact that most clinical vignettes in Step 1 will have classical presentations, but not always. But you need to understand the various ways the people who makes exam questions make the clinical vignette harder and what strategies you can use to overcome this.

It would be simpler if there is a step by step procedure you can follow to diagnose clinical vignettes. However, that would require that clinical vignettes follow a certain pattern. But you will encounter different variations in clinical vignettes so you need to adjust your approach accordingly.

First, there is the **direct approach.** The questions give you some signs and symptoms. Give you the diagnosis then ask the question. Yes, this happens in the USMLE, but you guessed it, not very often.

Second is the **simple approach**. You are given signs and symptoms of the patients that are relevant to the case at hand. Again diagnosis is usually straightforward in this case.

Third is the **pertinent positive and pertinent negative approach**. The questions give both signs and symptoms and absence of signs and symptoms that are relevant to the case are given and diagnosis is straightforward.

The next few approaches start making the clinical vignettes tougher, but only in appearance.

Fourth, the **"you need to interpret signs and symptoms" approach**. The questions this time do not give you signs and symptoms. Instead it gives you a patient description of his symptoms or a description of the signs you see. So you need to interpret these signs and symptoms first. Also it could just give you laboratory data with numbers and you need to interpret them first. Diagnosis seems more difficult but in reality is not because once you interpret the data, diagnosis is straightforward.

Fifth, the **irrelevant data approach**. The questions are usually long. It not only contains pertinent positives and negatives, but also contains irrelevant positive or negatives. This type of question is harder since you have to decide which signs and symptoms are relevant to the case and which are not. But it still is not that difficult because you will find later that only one possible disease can fit the diagnosis.

Now the next approach starts making the clinical vignette

harder.

Sixth, the **"barely enough data" approach**. The questions give you only very few signs and symptoms to diagnose the disease. It does not give all the classical signs and symptoms, just a few of them. This makes it harder to diagnose the case, because absence of some symptoms or signs you are expecting may throw you off the diagnosis. However, if you realize that you don't really have to have all the signs and symptoms to make a diagnosis and better yet know the minimum signs and symptoms you need to make a diagnosis, it's not impossible to diagnose this case. A good example will be a case of temporal arteritis in a middle-aged male. You expect the patient to be an old female, but it can happen in a younger male or female.

Seventh, the **"differentiate between two closely related diseases" approach**. The question focus on giving you pertinent but incomplete data that are the same for two closely related disease but makes sure it only contains one at most two details that can differentiate the disease. A good example is Crohn's Disease vs. Ulcerative Colitis. If you miss the crucial difference you will fail to diagnose the disease. Even if there are over a dozen differences, the question will only mention one or two. That's what makes it hard.

The other approaches are variations of the sixth and seventh approach. Combining the fourth and fifth approach to questions that uses the sixth and seventh approach makes the clinical vignette harder to diagnose.

So, how do we tackle these various types of clinical vignettes questions? Well basically we follow a few principles when dealing with clinical vignettes.

First, always rephrase the questions in your own words. A lot of times the wording of the question is what makes it complicated. By rephrasing the question, you simplify it. Also if you can't rephrase the question, you may not have understood it.

Second, interpret signs and symptoms and laboratory data if the question does not do so. You can even write it down on the writing materials provided for you in the exam. This way, it's easier to come up with a diagnosis.

Third, differentiate between positive signs and negative signs. Again you can use the writing materials provided and make two columns.

Fourth, decide if there are irrelevant data included. If you did the third step above, it's just a matter of crossing out positives and negatives not relevant to the case.

Fifth, if you have practiced diagnosing clinical vignettes as outlined in the how to study section, then you will be very familiar with the classical signs and symptoms of diseases and you can recognize patterns already. However, sometimes the pattern does not completely fit because of the sixth and seventh approach cited above or the adding of too much irrelevant data. The first step you need to do in this case is to decide if there are other cases that can fit the pattern. If not then the one that fits most closely, even incomplete is most probably the right answer.

If however, you realize that more than one disease can fit the pattern, then you may be dealing with a case that you need to differentiate. Understand that there may only be one or two details that differentiate the two. That is part of the reason why you are told to differentiate between concepts right from the start of this course. If you can't recall it, then the approach may be to look at the choices. Choices in the list may reflect one diagnosis over the other in which case, that is the diagnosis. Or it may contain choices that occur in either or both diagnosis, that makes it even harder and you may now have to guess.

Following the above principles will increase your chances of diagnosing clinical vignettes. But the only sure way to do so is to really master the clinical signs and symptoms of various diseases and to always make the extra step of differentiating between them throughout your review. ■

CHAPTER 78

SPEED BUILDING

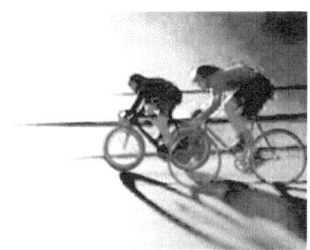

Why You Need to Do Speed Building Exercise

One of the most common complaints in the forums about this exam is how it is too long and how time is too short. A lot of people fail to finish all the questions in a block. And that can impact your score really badly. And yet you will be surprised at how many people don't even bother to train themselves, to answer questions faster.

One of the most common responses I get about speed building is this. 'I can go fast if I want to.' My answer is that everyone can go faster if they consciously try to do it. But if you are concentrating on going through questions faster, you are not concentrating on the questions and thinking about the answer. Once you start concentrating on the questions again, your speed goes down. You must make going through questions fast a habit. Not something you need to concentrate on. And habit requires time and practice.

Another thing you have to consider is that Step 1 is a 7

hour exam with 7 blocks. By the time you are doing the 5th or 6th block, your brain is turning to mush. You are tired. It takes you twice as long to think of answers. You have to read questions twice to understand them. Sometimes your mind just refuses to work and you have to close your eyes a minute or so to rest just to keep it functioning. So if you can barely finish the first block on time, you will never finish the later blocks. In my case, I finish my first block in 27 minutes. I finished my last block in 55 minutes. It's not because the last block is harder than the first, it's just my mind is too tired to function well. Also it does not mean that when I finished the first block in 27 minutes, I close the block. I spent all the extra time reviewing my answers.

How to Do Speed Building Exercise

In order to do speed building exercise, you need a computer based q bank to practice on. It is not recommended that you use one of the online q bank for this purpose. However, with the advent of additional online q banks outside of the big two, Kaplan and USMLE World, it can be an option. However, it is still best to use older q banks. The reason is that during speed building you are more concerned about answering questions fast then getting the answers right. Eventually as you get used to answering questions fast, your score will go higher.

When I started my own speed building exercise, I was scoring only in the 50's. After two months, I was hitting the 70's with occasional 80's. By the time I started with my online q banks, I was finishing a block in 35 minutes on average and scoring high 70's to low 80's.

In the course, there is speed building software that you can download from the site. You start downloading and using the software during your second revision. Alternatives you can use if you are not in the course include the Rapid Review Test

Materials. Just make sure the material is computer based. It does not have to have USMLE like questions. We have the online q banks for that.

You need to average one question every 15 seconds or 4 per minute. Initially do 15 minute daily drills doing 60 questions in the process. Then expand to 30 min doing 120 questions, eventually to one hour doing 240 questions. Your score will initially be terrible as mine was. But it will get better as you get used to going through questions very fast.

One of my students started out unable to finish all the questions in the block. On average he will miss 5 to 7 questions per block. 6 weeks after speed building practice, he was finishing each block on average in 45 minutes and got a 92 eventually. ■

CHAPTER 79

UNDERSTANDING HOW QUESTIONS ARE CONSTRUCTED

Why You Need to Know How Questions are Constructed

Whenever I discuss about how to answer questions with my students, I am surprised at how little they know about how questions are constructed. This is evident in the questions they ask or certain presuppositions they have. For example, sometimes they will justify why their wrong answer is valid because of one detail in the question. But if you know how questions are constructed, you know sometimes they add one tiny detail to throw you off and therefore you need to decide if that tiny detail is enough to change the answer. Of course sometimes that one tiny detail can affect the answer.

Even the answer choices are dictated a lot of time by how the question is constructed. And if you are able to see how the choices were derived at, it can help you get to the right answer. Or at minimum help you decide how to approach the question to find the answers.

Also understanding how questions are constructed can help you in your review. I always tell my students that whenever they finish studying a concept or integrating a concept in their review, they should ask themselves this, ' how would I make a question about this concept?' This will not only help you solidify what you know about the concept, but even help you anticipate possible questions that may come out. Also knowing techniques in question construction can help you anticipate the variations of a question that can appear in the exam.

How are Questions Constructed and How they are Made Tougher

The following steps describe how questions are commonly constructed. Not all questions pass through all the steps and there may be other variations on these methods.

First understand that basically most questions you encounter will primarily be of three types:

1. *Tell me what you know, or basically what you have memorized.*

2. *Differentiate between two concepts, which form the bulk of Step 1 questions*

3. *Given or knowing A and B what is C?*

Then these basic questions are made tougher by some modifications.

- **Asking them in clinical vignette format.** This requires you to make a diagnosis first before you can answer the question.

- **You need to interpret signs, symptoms and laboratory.** Instead of giving you the signs and symptoms outright, it describes the signs and symptoms to you or gives you the numbers or description of laboratory results.

- **Irrelevant data is included** and it's up to you to decide which data is relevant and which is not. Some people make the mistake of always presuming all the data given is significant. On the other hand incorrectly ignoring significant data can harm you.

- **They start with all answer choices being correct answers, and then alter all the other choices slightly until only one answer is correct.** Therefore, all the answers may look correct, or may only be slightly wrong except for one answer.

- **The choices require you to think from multiple contexts to come up with the correct answer.**

- **The choices require two to three step thinking in order to be able to find the answer.** So unless you know the direct answer, it is harder to chain facts together to arrive at a right answer.

- **The choices contain distractors.** Distractors are usually based on common medical misconceptions, words with the same pronunciation or nearly the same pronunciation but different meaning, a previous medical fact that is now obsolete.

- **Asking very low yield topics.** There are always a few very low yield topic coming out and the sole purpose is to rattle you.

To Illustrate a Type 1 Question will look like this:

Which one of the following laboratory determination is abnormal in Idiopathic Thrombocytopenic Purpura?

- APTT

- BT*

- CT

- PT

- TT

You will notice that the question is straightforward. If you know what laboratory abnormality occurs in ITP, which is prolonged bleeding time, then you got the answer.

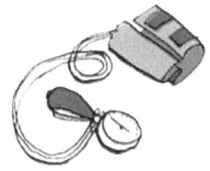

A Type II question will look like this.

This is a case of a 48 year old male with poorly controlled hypertension for the past 2 years. For the past 3 months the patients BP has been greater than 260/130 and the patients serum creatinine is increased indicating malignant hypertension. What vascular lesion do you expect in the kidney?

1.   Hyperplastic arteriolosclerosis*

2.   Granulomatous arteritis

3.   Hyaline arteriolosclerosis

4.   Necrotizing vasculitis

5.   Medial calcific sclerosis

Answering this question is fairly straightforward. First so long as you know what vascular lesions occur in the kidney in hypertension, you are good. In this case it's 1 and 3, with the rest having nothing to do with hypertension. If you had reviewed by organizing the topics in your head you would have arrived at this point pretty fast. Narrow down the topic, any choices not related to the topic, eliminate.

The next step you need to differentiate between the two types of vascular lesions in the kidney caused by hypertension. If you had taken the steps to differentiate between concepts during your prep as you were instructed from the start, this would not be a problem. The two lesions occur in two different circumstances in hypertension. Hyperplastic arteriolosclerosis occurs in cases of malignant hypertension while hyaline arteriolosclerosis occurs in longstanding poorly controlled hypertension. While the patient's hypertension is poorly controlled, he is now in malignant hypertension due to the high BP and evidence of end-organ failure with elevated serum creatinine.

Once you know how to differentiate between poorly controlled hypertension and malignant hypertension answering this question is again fairly straightforward. I hope you are noticing a pattern we are using to arrive at answers. And how studying the way I have advocated from the start can help you arrive at the answer much more quickly.

Let's take a look at a Type III question. The example I am using is matching type which accounts for 10% of the question in each block.

Match the clinical condition to the etiologic factor.

1. Localized radiation treatment of Cancer - E, F

2. Acute total body radiation of 300 rad - B

3. Acute total body radiation of 1000 rad - C

4. Acute total body radiation of 2000 rad - D

5. Survivor of atomic bomb explosion - A

A. Leukemia

B. Hematopoietic failure in 2 weeks

C. Death due to GI syndrome in 3 days

D. CNS symptoms within hours

E. Fibrosing pneumonitis

F. Radio dermatitis

This question requires some analysis to answer. This is actually a question in the online quiz for my online pathology course. Too often students will complain that they can't google for the answer. In questions of this type, the tester is trying to see if you can make conclusions based on certain facts that you know. It tests your analytical skill. If the answer can be googled, it becomes a test of your memorization skill.

Of course to be able to answer this question you need to know some facts. First you need to know the effects of chronic low dose radiation exposure. Second, the chronic effect of an acute non-lethal dose radiation exposure. And lastly, the relative radiosensitivity of various tissues of the human body.

Looking at the first etiologic factor, we know the patient is undergoing chronic low dose exposure to radiation. Choice A is a possible answer, but choice B, C and D are due to acute radiation poisoning. Choice E and F are also possible answers. Looking at etiologic factor 2, 3 and 4, we note they are all acute radiation exposure and therefore it seems choices B, C and D are their matches. Meanwhile the 5th etiologic factor causes sublethal dose of radiation. And as a survivor he is probably suffering from a condition that arises years after the exposure. Therefore choice A, Leukemia seems to be the best choice. Meanwhile choice E and F are both due to chronic low dose exposure to radiation which occurs in low dose radiation treatment for cancer, so factor 1 is matched with choice E and F.

That leaves us with factor 2, 3 and 4, all acute radiation exposure of different degree to be paired with B, C and D, all clinical conditions caused by acute radiation exposure of different magnitudes. The key to answering this part is knowing radiosensitivity of various tissues of the human body. The three tissues involved are hematopoietic, gastrointestinal and CNS tissues. Hematopoietic tissues are most radiosensitve, followed by GI, then CNS being the most radioresistant. Therefore, hematopoietic failure in two weeks compared to CNS effects within hours indicate the first condition to be due to a relatively low dose exposure while CNS effect within hours indicate a very high dose of exposure. Meanwhile, GI effects in 3 days show intermediate level of exposure.

Therefore looking at the factors, we can now match 300 rad exposure(2) to hematopoietic failure(B), 1000 rad exposure(3) to GI failure(C) and 2000 rad exposure(4) to CNS effects(D).

As you can see, answering this question is possible by knowing a few facts and using analytical skills to arrive at an answer. Type III questions are not too numerous in Step 1 accounting for anywhere between 10 to 20% of the questions.

We will now give a few examples of how these questions are made tougher. We cannot discuss all the variation in detail as it will require giving dozens of examples which are too big for this text or lecture to cover. We will discuss them during the test preparation phase in the course when we do group analysis exercise and discussion about questions. It's called 'How would you go about answering this question?' sessions. Each student is asked to explain why he or she chose a certain answer and the thought process involved. It emphasizes the process rather than getting the actual question right as a lot of times you can get the right answer with a lucky guess.

An example of the Type I question transformed to a clinical vignette question looks like this.

This is a case of a 38 year old female with several months' history of nose bleed, easy bruisability and increased bleeding with menses. There are no other complaints. Physical examination shows scattered petechiae. Peripheral smear shows decreased platelets, normal RBC morphology. Meanwhile, bone marrow biopsy shows increased megakaryocytes. Which one of the following laboratory determination is abnormal in the above case?

1. APTT
2. BT*
3. CT
4. PT
5. TT

This is exactly the same case as the first one. Except it now requires you to recognize this as a case of ITP rather than telling you outright that it is one. It requires more analysis and if you fail to diagnose it, you can't answer the question. This is actually an easy clinical vignettes as it gives you the signs and symptoms outright. it could have given you descriptions rather than actual findings. For example stating that menses lasts for 7 days and averaging 8 napkins a day rather than the usual 5 days and 4 napkins per day. Describing the petechiae as rashes that do not blanch with pressure. Giving you the actual platelet count while describing the actual RBC morphology. All this will increase the toughness of the question although it still is basically the same question.

Of course the correct strategy to employ is to simplify the question. First you need to diagnose the case. Start by interpreting the signs and symptoms as required. Recognize the pattern and diagnose the case. The question now becomes simply a case of ITP and the laboratory abnormality noted.

Another way to increase the toughness of the question is to fiddle with the answer choices. Take a look at this example. It's the same question as before but we now change the answer choices.

Which one of the following pattern of laboratory determination is typical in the above case?

1. Normal APTT, normal BT, normal PT

2. Normal APTT, normal PT, abnormal BT*

3. Abnormal APTT, normal BT, abnormal PT

4. Abnormal APTT, abnormal BT, normal PT

5. Abnormal APTT, abnormal PT, abnormal BT

Whereas in the first case it only requires you to think which laboratory test is abnormal, presenting the answer choices this way now requires you think not only in the context of which tests are normal and which tests are abnormal, you need to decide what pattern of abnormalities will appear. This effectively makes the question more, complex. In reality, it is still the same simple question as the first one. Knowing that only bleeding time is abnormal and the rest normal make it easy to choose number 2. However, if like most people, you tend to choose the answer from the choices rather than deciding on the answer immediately after reading the question, the choices can momentarily confuse you.

Throughout the course, you are being asked to study a certain way, to acquire certain ways in your approach to answering questions. The reasons are it helps you counter all the test maker's effort to make the question tougher. By following the study methods taught in the course, we try to anticipate these tactics used by test makers to toughen the exam and counter them, thereby minimizing their negative effect on our ability to get the right answer.

Now let's look at a type II question being made tougher in clinical vignette format. It also requires you to interpret signs and symptoms.

This is a case of a 48 year old male with a 10 year history of BP ranging from 155/100 to 165/110. The past 3 months BP rose to 260/130. Patient complains of occasional headaches. Other vital signs include PR: 70/min, RR: 14/min. Laboratory findings include: FBS 100 mg/dL, creatinine 3.9 mg/dL, BUA 5 mg/dL, Na 140 mmol/L, and K,4.5 mmol/L. Urinalysis are as follows, pH: 6.0, SG: 1.015, sugar (-), protein (T), bacteria: +++, WBC: 0-2/hpf, RBC: 0-1/hpf, hyaline casts: 0-1/hpf. What vascular lesion do you expect in the kidney?

1. Hyperplastic arteriolosclerosis*

2. Granulomatous arteritis

3. Hyaline arteriolosclerosis

4. Necrotizing vasculitis

5.   Medial calcific sclerosis

This question is actually the same as the original Type II question. But here you have to diagnose the clinical vignette. You need to know that this person has longstanding poorly controlled hypertension and has gone into malignant hypertension already. Take note that a lot of insignificant data both positive and negative is included. Again if you were unable to diagnose this clinical vignette, then you will miss the answer completely.

Now another way to make the question more difficult is to tweak the answer choices. The two most common methods are the use of two-to-three step thinking choices and distractors. Let's look at an example below.

What vascular lesion do you expect in the kidney?

1.   Marked laminated "onion-skin" thickening of the arteriolar walls.*

2.   Fibrinoid necrosis of small arteries and early infiltration by neutrophils with subsequent fibrosis and granuloma formation.

3.   Hyaline thickening of the arteriolar walls.

4.   Destruction of the arterial media and internal elastic lamella of arteries.

5.   Ring-like calcification in the media of arteries.

Here instead of the original pathologic term of the vascular lesion, you find a description of the lesion. In order to be able to answer this question, you need first to know the vascular lesion involved before you can associate it with the description of the vascular lesion. This is an example of a two-step thinking question. This happens because we don't associate the description of hyperplastic arteriolosclerosis with malignant hypertension. Instead with associate the term hyperplastic arteriosclerosis with malignant hypertension. Same thing we don't associate the clinical signs and symptoms of malignant hypertension with hyperplastic arteriolosclerosis but with the term malignant hypertension itself. This makes it easier to memorize them.So you could say clinical vignettesis a form of two-step thinking question already. So with the clinical vignette and description on the lesions you are technically dealing with a three step thinking question.

The same holds true when dealing with treatment. You first have to diagnose the case, then the treatment. One more step is when the choices involve side effects of the treatment of choice rather than the treatment. So this chain of facts could go on for a long while. Again the best way to tackle questions like this is to anticipate them and do your own chaining during the review. Don't just memorize say malignant hypertension -> hyperplastic arteriosclerosis. Instead go all the way. Clinical signs and symptoms -> malignant hypertension -> hyperplastic arteriolosclerosis -> description of lesion. It pays to know the clinical description of every buzzword.

How This Knowledge Helps You to Answer Questions Better

First, understand that a lot of simple questions exist in the USMLE and they only look tough when they are modified as indicated above. If you are able to see the methods they use to make a question tougher, you can simplify the question better and increase your chance of getting the right answer. Although how well you are able to detect these methods and the total number of questions you can simplify depends a lot on your intelligence, even if you are only able to do this on 10% of the questions that is 10% more questions you got right or finished faster. Even I wasn't able to break down all the questions this way, but it was doable for about 40 to 50% of the questions for me.

Second, by understanding how questions are made tougher, you can prepare for them ahead during your prep. Study clinical vignettes. Know how to interpret symptoms, signs and laboratory data. Know the actual description of all buzzwords. Always try to know what is relevant to a particular topic. This can be done by topic organization. If most of the data is consistent with one topic, it's a clue that those not consistent may be irrelevant. Learn how to deal with distractors and questions requiring two to three step thinking. Understand especially when doing online q banks, that some of those questions deal with very low yield topics, so take it in stride and don't panic.■

CHAPTER 80
ANALYZING QUESTIONS

If you want to get a good score, one of the most important skills you need to acquire is to learn how to analyze questions. There are various reasons why it will help you score better and we will discuss them a little while. However, the best way to learn how to do it is by discussing questions after you have gone through it yourself. It is a completely different process from what most people do when they read the explanations to answers after they finished answering q banks. Those explanations tell you why an answer is factually right and why all the other choices are factually wrong.

However, most problems you have when you start answering questions are how to get to the right answer. How many times has it happened that once you see the correct answer, you know it's correct and your choice is wrong without even reading the explanations yet? Therefore, the problem is why did you wind up choosing the wrong answer even if you know what the answer is. Or why were you down to last two choices when apparently the right answer seems obvious in hindsight? The answer lies in your thought process and how you analyzed the question. Good test writers are able to take advantage of the way we think, write a simple question in a more complicated manner and fool us into choosing the wrong answer. That is in essence what a tough question is. And the only way to counter that is superior analytical skills.

Why Question Analysis Will Help You Score Higher?

There are a lot of ways to approach a question and analyze it so your chance of arriving at a correct answer is higher. Too many times people have complained that they know the topic asked by the question and even the answer but wind up choosing the wrong answer. A lot of times they even blame wrong analysis as the culprit, but usually concluding that they over analyzed the question. This usually means they got faked by the question to choose the wrong answer.

The best way to learn how to analyze questions is by answering questions and discussing the thought process involved in your analysis. The correct factual answer is secondary. Of course in the actual exam, both are important. In training your analytical skills, getting the correct answer by wrong analysis or luck is not acceptable. Therefore, this is best done in group discussions.

In the course, once you start doing q banks, you join regular sessions discussing questions where you present your thought process in coming up with the answer. You compare your thought process with others and decide which is the best approach. I will then put in my two cents worth. I do not claim to be correct in all cases as previous students have shown me a thing or two about superb analysis. So in the process we learn from each other.

Just discussing the different analytical approach in analysis is not very effective in learning this skill. The most effective way is going over your own thought process and comparing it with others. Therefore, I will just give a few examples and the rest you should learn during discussion sessions.

The first steps in improving your ability to analyze questions are to learn how tough questions are constructed, and the different ways clinical vignettes can be presented. Please refer to appropriate sections in this chapter for details.

One of the most common technique test makers do to fake you into choosing the wrong answer is to give you two opposite condition and then ask you which of the statement is true or not true given one of the condition. In this case it is very important to make sure you understand which condition is being referred to and whether it is asking for a true statement or not. Too many people get the wrong answer because they fail to catch this trick.

For example, given a patient who came into the ER after an automobile accident, your examination finds him to be in a state of shock. Remember this could be in the form of a clinical vignette. Then it states that you gave him 2 L of Lactated Ringer's solution over an hour. Immediately you think, the patient is hydrated. You should be very careful when you read the question. A lot of people get faked by presuming the patient is already on a hydrated state. The question may turn around and ask what condition is prevalent in the patient before you rehydrated him. The choices given will be either pathophysiologic condition in the dehydrated patient or in the rehydrated patient. Being alert with this type of question can minimize the chance you get faked by them.

There are a lot of other types of questions that can appear in the exam and learning how to analyze questions is important to score high. It is too numerous to discuss here, but will be discuss in the 'How would you answer this question?' sessions in the course proper. ■

CHAPTER 81

STRATEGIES FOR ANSWERING QUESTIONS ON THE DAY OF THE EXAM

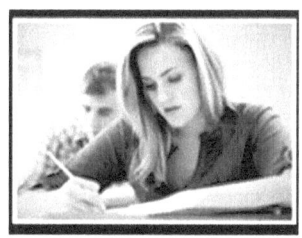

On the day of the exam, how you go about answering the questions can impact your score a lot. Although there are many things you can do to increase your chances of getting the correct answer on exam day during your prep, what you do on exam day is still the most crucial factor that will affect how well you do in the exam.

First, always go as fast as you can. This is where a lot of test-takers make a mistake and a big one at that. This is partially because most prep courses, reviewers and forums seem to recommend that since you have on average about 80 seconds to answer each question, it is alright to spend more or less that amount of time on each question. Nothing can be more disastrous. There are a lot of tough questions in the USMLE and believe me, it will take more than 80 seconds to answer them.

The correct strategy is to go through easy questions as fast as you can. If you can answer a question in 20 seconds why spend 80 seconds on it. Save those extra seconds for answering tough questions. Therefore, you need to train yourself to go through questions fast.

Second, always think of the answer before you look at the choices. A big reason why distractors and two to three step thinking questions are effective is our bad habit of looking for the answers in the choices rather than thinking of the answer immediately after reading the question stem.

Distractors are two answer choices that are almost the same. This serves to confuse you on what the right answer is. By thinking of the answer first, then the answer choice nearest to the answer you thought of is the most likely correct answer. This tends to minimize the effect of distractors.

Two-to-three step thinking questions make it harder for you to pick the right answer as you need to chain together multiple related facts before you can pick the correct answer choice. This can be confusing. By thinking of the answer before you see the choices, you have an idea of the answer you are looking for and will also tend to shorten the length of the chain of facts you need to put together to get the answer choices.

Of course, you can't always think of the answer without looking at the answer choices. But the more questions you are able to do that, the better the chance that you will get more correct answers.

Third, always rephrase and simplify the question. A lot of times, questions are made more difficult due to wordiness or the use of complicated language. By rephrasing questions and simplifying them in the process, you will find that what seems like a difficult question is actually quite straightforward.

Also,by rephrasing a question, you insure that you really understood the question. A lot of times people chose the wrong answer because they misunderstood the question. Rephrasing it in your own words helps insure that you have understood the question.

Fourth, never leave a question blank. One of the biggest reason people fail this exam is that they fail to answer all the questions in the exam. That is the main reason why part of the test preparation phase emphasizes doing speed building exercise in doing questions. It helps train you to go through questions and increase your speed of recalling random information. If you had followed that advice you should have no problem finishing your questions.

The USMLE is a multiple choice type of question. Which means that at least one of the answer choices is correct. Therefore make sure every question is answered even if you are only guessing, or you are just picking answers at random because you have run out of time. There is a detailed discussion on a systematic way of doing this on the section on What to Do on the Day of the Exam.

Fifth, stick to your first choice unless there is a compelling reason to change your answer. Statistics show that when you are not sure of your answer and choosing between two choices, >50% of the time your first choice will be correct, while your second choice will only be correct < 50% of the time. I know the difference is very small but there is still a difference. Therefore, change your answer only when there is a compelling reason to do so.

What can be considered compelling reasons? One is that you are definitely sure that your first answer is wrong. The statistics above apply only if you are unsure which of the two is correct. Another is that you misread or misunderstood the question when you chose your first answer. And now that you understood it, the second choice is the better answer. Then you can change it.

Sixth, spend a maximum of 2 minutes on a hard question. If you had followed the first instruction noted above, then you would now have more time to answer really tough question. However, the extra time you have is finite, so you still have to use them wisely. Remember that in the USMLE, each question is worth one point. It does not matter if it's easy or hard, it still is worth one point. So spending too much time on a hard question and missing easy questions in the process is not really a good strategy.

So spend a maximum of two minutes even on a hard question. If you still can't get an answer or are down to last two choices, then pick one and move on. Spending more than that amount of time rarely results in a better answer, although it still can happen. Just mark the question and come back to it once you have finished the block and you have more time left.

Seventh, once you have finished answering a question, forget it and move to the next one. Always concentrate on the question at hand. One of the biggest temptation, especially on questions we have spent a long time thinking through or down to last two is to continue thinking about it even if we have moved to the next question. The problem in doing that is that we are not concentrating on the question at hand but on the previous question. This increases the chance that you can get the present question wrong even if it's a relatively easy question. Therefore it is important to forget the previous question and concentrate on the question you are answering now. Just mark the previous question, come back to it later if you have time.

The same thing holds through after you finish one block and have moved on to another. Forget about the previous block and concentrate on the block you are currently answering. You cannot change any answer in the previous block. Worrying about it will not increase your score. In fact it may even lower your score since it distracts you from concentrating on the block you are answering and increases your chance of getting things wrong. ■

***

unit 12

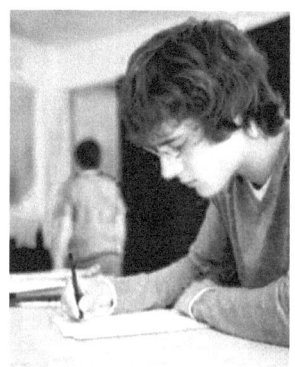

What to Do on the Day of the Exam

CHAPTER 82

INTRODUCTION

The USMLE Step 1 is perhaps one of the toughest exams you will face in your professional life. Therefore, you need to be well-prepared for this exam. This exam is difficult for the following reasons:

First, it covers a tremendous amount of material and yet you need to remember all of them for that one day in the exam. You also need to be able to recall them fast.

Second, it is a very long exam. The exam covers 8 hours. 7 hours of exam time and 1 hour of break time. It is very exhausting and fatigue can affect your score tremendously.

Third, as far as the USMLE is concerned, what you cannot remember, in a minute or less, you do not know. Even if you studied them, you get no partial points. You may study for months, but everything depends on that one day you sit for the exam.

So, it is very important that you are at your best on the day of the examination. And preparations to be at your best on the day of the exam starts weeks before the actual exam day.

Basically, one of the most important enemies you need to fight is ***stress***. Step 1 by itself is a very stressful exam. So you need to minimize all stresses that are not directly related to the exam. Stress is additive and adding unnecessary stress on the exam day itself will undo you. ■

CHAPTER 83

BE AT YOUR BEST ON THE DAY OF THE USMLE EXAM

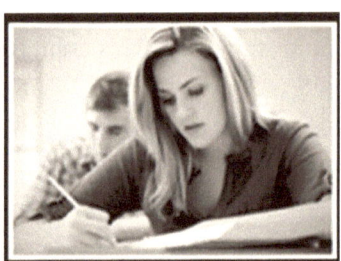

So what do you do on the day of the USMLE examination? The day you sit for the USMLE is the culmination of months of preparation. It may seem unfair that no matter how well your performance were in those countless q banks and test simulation, the only performance that really counts is the one you do on exam day. Therefore, it makes sense to maximize your chances of performing well for that date.

Your preparation should begin way before the date of your USMLE examination, when you schedule the examination. It is a known fact that during review, people do reach a plateau and the best time to sit for the USMLE exam is just before or just after you reach your peak. Earlier or later than that can result in lower scores. During review, immediately after learning and memorizing your lessons, you start forgetting right away. Normally, the amount of medical concepts you are memorizing and retaining is growing faster than you are forgetting them.

However, there comes a time when you reach your peak and eventually plateau. Afterwards you will go into decline and forget more than you are learning. Most people go into plateau in about 6 to 8 months; therefore the ideal review time for the USMLE is around that long. That is why my USMLE Step 1 prep course is around 6 months long.

To be on your best on the day of the exam requires advanced planning. First, you need to be well-rested on the day of the exam. But you also need to be alert and on your toes. Second, you need to minimize all unnecessary stress on the day of the exam. The USMLE is a very stressful exam already; additional stress can wear you down and decrease your performance. Third, you need to be prepared for any contingency and plan for it. If nothing untoward happens, well and good, but if something does, you have a plan for it. ■

CHAPTER 84

STOP STUDYING FOR THE USMLE EXAM AT THE RIGHT TIME

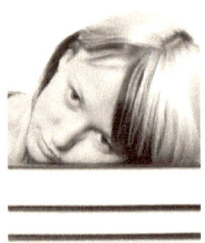

When I was doing my prep, it was really exhausting; the amount of material I needed to cover was tremendous. Q banks were exhausting and nerve-wracking at the same time. However, in order to be well rested on the day of the exam, you need to stop studying way before exam day or at least lighten up the load so you can rest.

So the question you have to ask yourself is when do you actually stop studying? Some make the mistake of studying right up to the night before they sit for the USMLE exam while others start relaxing two weeks before their scheduled USMLE exam.

What is wrong with studying up to the last minute? Well to illustrate, imagine a marathon runner who the day before the marathon decides to do a marathon to see if he can win the marathon. How well do you think they will perform when they run the actual marathon the next day? Badly, right? The USMLE is an exhausting exam that will test your stamina to the limit. Anyone who has taken the USMLE exam can tell you that their brains felt like mush and refuses to function properly in the last 2 blocks of the USMLE exam. I know, mine did. Plus after the exam, it took me two days to recover from the exhaustion. Therefore, it makes sense to rest as much as possible the day before the examination to regenerate your energy for the battle ahead. In fact I recommend to start lightening up your study schedule 2 weeks before the exam and to stop studying completely 2 days before the actual day of your USMLE examination.

Now if resting is good, why shouldn't I rest one or two weeks before my scheduled USMLE exam? Again, let's use a sports example to answer this question. Professional boxers usually arrive a week or 2 before the bout to the venue where the bout will be held. By this time they've already finished their training. Any boxer, who has not finished training for the bout by that time, is bound to lose the fight. And yet instead of painting the town red, they spend their time in the gym, practicing and sparring. The reason is so that they can maintain focus on the bout itself. Losing focus this late may mean losing the bout. The same holds true with preparing for the USMLE. The problem most old grads have is to start their USMLE review. They usually go through lots of false starts before their review start going smoothly. The main reason is that it's been too long since they've studied and there are lots of things going on in their life that it's hard to focus on the prep. Getting distracted and losing focus too early before the exam can cause you to perform at less than peak condition in the actual USMLE examination. You need to block off everything until you've finished the exam. ■

CHAPTER 85

WHAT TO DO LAST 2 WEEKS BEFORE THE ACTUAL USMLE EXAM

So what should you be doing starting 2 weeks before the actual examination? Well definitely you should have finished the heavy lifting and not studying anything new. The reason is that your mind will tend to remember better the most recent things you have studied and if that is low yield new stuff (presuming you studied the higher yield stuff first), that is what you will remember better and unfortunately has less chances of appearing in the exam. Therefore the best thing to do at this point is try to cover the highest yield stuff. If you are in my course, you would be enrolled in the High Yield Fast Facts (HYFF) Course, a compilation of the highest yield test materials in electronic flashcard format. If you are reviewing on your own, you can use the Rapid Review section of First Aid at the back of the book. However, it is in table format which is less effective than in flashcard format. This way you remember the highest yield information best when you sit for the exam. (Did I mention that someone who got a 99/256 use my HYFF course two weeks before the exam?)

You should also be doing only one to two blocks of q bank a day at this time. That is to keep you in top shape to answer questions. You should have finished simulating the exam before this time. The minimum simulation you need to do is four blocks. 2 blocks straight, 10 minute break, then 2 blocks straight again. But do this way before the last two weeks.

Another thing you should consider is your sleep-wake cycle. If you are a night owl, your peak performance tends to be at night and you wake up late in the morning. But the exam is during the day so you need to synchronize your cycle so you peak during the day. Sleep early and wake up early preferably the same time schedule as you need to sleep and wake up on the day of the exam. This way your body will tend to get used to the time you need to be at your peak during exam day. Plus if you sleep in the afternoon or take a nap, stop doing this two weeks before the exam. Or your body will get used to sleeping at the time when you should be wide awake answering questions. Lastly, do your q banks during the day and not at night again so you get used to answering questions during daytime.

Another important thing to consider is how far you lived from the Prometric Center where you will be taking your USMLE exam. The exam is a high stress event. If you have to drive through traffic and you are 2 hours away, the stress can be tremendous. Worse, traffic may be unpredictable and you may get there late. In my case, I lived about 1 hour by car from the Prometric exam site. The route I have to travel is notorious for unpredictable traffic that could last for 2 to 3 hours. So instead of increasing my own stress. I booked myself into a hotel about 10 minute walk from the site the night before. I could take a cab (parking is also terrible) and be there in about 3 minutes including traffic light change. And if for some reason, I couldn't get a cab or traffic is at a standstill, I could walk and be on the exam site in 10 minutes. US$100, the price of one night in the hotel is small compared to the $800++ exam fees, $1000++ for books, qbanks, NBME, etc. and 7 months of prep time I had already invested so far. Cab fare is $5 plus tip.

What to Do the Last 2 Days before the USMLE Exam

You can spend the last 2 days before the examination on anything to relax you. I watched a movie before my exam. A comedy, Ice Age 2. Please don't do any studying. Not even a high yield review. Your brain needs to be rested so it can function at peak condition on exam day.

Then on the night before the exam, the most important thing is to get a good night's rest. That involves a regular meal, not too heavy. Maybe a nice warm bath. Sleep early so you can wake up early. But do not take tranquilizers as that can cause you not to be in peak form the next day. Make sure everything you need is prepared beforehand. (Clothes, food, water, medicine, ID, Exam permit, etc.) Preparing it early in the morning just increases your stress level. In fact if you can prepare everything 2 days before so much the better.

Remember, stress is additive. The USMLE examination itself is an extremely stressful event. Any other worries on the same day just add to the stress. So prepare everything at least 2 to 3 days beforehand so that your only worry is the examination itself on that crucial day. ■

CHAPTER 86

WHAT TO DO ON THE DAY OF THE EXAMINATION

Now, a few things to remember on the day of the examination itself: The most important is to ***never leave a question blank.*** There is no penalty for a wrong answer. The USMLE is an MCQ exam and one answer is always correct. An unanswered question is a sure wrong, while a question answered even with a guess is a possible right. And just one additional right answer may mean the difference between a 74 and 75 or a 98 and 99. As sports great Wayne Gretzky said, "You miss 100% of the shot you do not take."

So what's a method to make sure you do this? Well, you should allocate around 10 seconds per question to randomly pick the answer once your time runs out. At the two minute warning, it means you can randomly answer at least 12 questions. So if you have less than that to answer then you can start randomly answering the questions that you have not finished. For example at the 2 minute warning, you have six questions unanswered. Continue answering as before, but at the one minute mark, just randomly guess an answer on the remaining unanswered questions.

Now for pacing in the actual examination: The best pacing schedule makes use of a couple of facts. One, you are more alert in the early morning than in the afternoon when the exam will have taken its toll. Therefore it makes sense to schedule more blocks before lunch. So for USMLE Step 1, 4, 3 would be good. Now you are sleepiest after lunch, because of the act of digestion, therefore schedule only 1 block after lunch then have a break afterward. Never take more than 2 blocks before you take a break with some food or sugared drink. Your sugar level starts falling after 2 hours (physiology of fasting) and sugar is the main fuel for your brain.

So best to schedule 2 blocks, 15 minute break, 2 blocks then 25 minute lunch, then 1 block, 10 minute break, then last 2 blocks. You can take a break between the last 2 blocks if you feel you need it. Notice that the total break is 50 minutes. Reason is that the actual break will usually be longer than the time you scheduled it. Just logging in and out of the room will take 1.5 to 2 minutes. The rest room is usually two doors out (both the exam center in my home country and the one in San Francisco where I took Step 3 have the same layout. So I presume all Prometric centers have the same general layout) So you have to walk a bit. If you just need a short break between blocks, just sit on your cubicle and rest for a minute or two before starting the next block. As I said logging in and out is a time waster.

Scheduling Meals and Breaks on the Day of the USMLE Exam

Now we need to talk about scheduling meals and breaks and what to eat. Light breakfast in the morning preferably no meat but high energy carbohydrate. (High protein, high fat foods can make you sleepy, so no ham and eggs, sorry) Now coffee or tea to keep you awake, but limit to a cup since they increase urine formation.(increased heart rate, increased GFR = increased urine formation)

For the morning break, do not bring sandwich. It takes too long to finish eating it. Bring something sweet, high energy, high carbohydrate that can give you a sugar boost. (I ate a small high sugar cake that I finished in 4 to 5 bites.) You can opt to wash down with a cola (which can provide both sugar and caffeine boost) Do not skip the morning break. Remember your brain needs sugar to function properly. For the USMLE exam, you need your brain to function at peak condition.

For lunch break, do not eat a full meal. A sandwich, preferably not high protein (egg sandwich or cheese sandwich comes to mind) is advisable. It's actually basic physiology. A heavy meal will cause blood flow to be diverted to your GI tract longer therefore less blood flow to brain. Plus, proteins and fat will cause secretion of more HCl for digestion leading to Metabolic alkalosis. This leads to hypoventilation (to increase CO_2) and therefore less oxygen to the brain. Longer digestive time causes longer time for HCl to be reabsorbed. This is the main reason why you are sleepiest after lunch.

For the afternoon break, a high sugary drink whether cola or juice will suffice. Limit total water intake as that can increase need for bathroom breaks.(600 to 800 ml will be enough, max 2 breaks)

Medicines You might Need on the Day of the USMLE Exam

- Now for the meds, you need the following.

- Pain reliever - paracetamol, in case of headache or any other ache.

- Loperamide - in case of gastrointestinal emergency eg. diarrhea

- Antacid - in case of hyperacidity (anxiety can cause it

- Beta blocker - in case anxiety and palpitation become too distracting.

Don't forget to bring any other meds you may need (anti-histamine if you have allergies, salbutamol inhaler if you are asthmatic, etc.)

Last Words

Now one last word of advice. Once you finish a block, forget about it. Concentrate on the block you are currently answering. Worrying about a block you have finished will not raise your score. Concentrating on the current block will help raise your score. Not paying attention to your current block because you are busy worrying about the previous block will even lower your score.

After you finish the exam. Go home. Stop thinking about the exam. Have dinner with your family, whom you probably haven't spoken to in months. Then take on a week-long vacation before even starting to worry about your USMLE score. In the meantime, prepare what you want to write on the exam experience page of your favorite forum. ■

***

ABOUT THE AUTHOR

Mike Nicol Uy, MD also known as *askdoc* in the USMLE Prep Community is founder & CEO of askdoc-usmle.com. He has been teaching people how to prep for the USMLE since 2008 and have helped hundreds pass this exam. He took his Step 1 and Step 2CK in 2006 and scored 99/256 & 99/258, respectively. He passed the USMLE Step 2 CS and Step 3 in 2007 with a score of 90/219. You can contact him at his blog: **http://blogs.askdoc-usmle.com**

www.ingramcontent.com/pod-product-compliance
Lightning Source LLC
Chambersburg PA
CBHW031817170526
45157CB00001B/90